Financial Strategies for Physicians

Paul H. Sutherland, CFP
Financial and Investment Management Group
Suttons Bay, Michigan

Grune & Stratton, Inc.

Harcourt Brace Jovanovich, Publishers

Philadelphia   New York   San Diego   London
San Francisco   Tokyo   Sydney   Toronto

Grune & Stratton, Inc.
West Washington Square
Philadelphia, Pennsylvania 19105

Distributed in the United Kingdom by
Grune & Stratton, Ltd.
24/28 Oval Road, London NW 1

International Standard Book Number   0-8089-1831-1
Printed in the United States of America
88 89 90 91   10 9 8 7 6 5 4 3 2 1

Dedication

Dale E. Sutherland

Father, mentor, and friend.

Acknowledgments

Special thanks must go to Robert Feigenbaum, my editor at *Physician's Management* for catalyzing this project and introducing me to my editors at Harcourt Brace Jovanovich, Publishers, Grune & Stratton, Inc.

I started toying with the idea of a book on financial planning for physicians 4 years ago and with Bob Feigenbaum's encouragement, I was able to get started.

I appreciate the support of my wife, Kimberly, who gave me the freedom and support to pursue this project.

Without the help of my secretary, Linda Brzezinski's candid editorial assistance, intuitive ability to read my handwriting, and positive attitude, I don't know how I would have completed *Financial Strategies for Physicians*.

Others who helped directly and indirectly in this project were Annabelle McIlnay, freelance writer from Detroit; Mary W. Sutherland; Terry Rogers, tax attorney, Traverse City, Michigan; David Kerr, attorney; Robert P. Coleman, C.P.A.; insurance professionals James Day, Steve Grinnell, David A. Creamer, Harry Wiberg, and Hal Lyman; Jesse R. Gillett, C.P.A.; money managers Charles Royce, Harvey Eisen, Robert Jeavons, Joseph N. Pecoraro, and Allen Lancz. Special thanks to my colleague and associate, Jeff K. Pasche, who said he didn't mind late night phone calls to discuss the chapters on investment management and for his help with research.

Barbara Graves, Carol Milmine, and Harold W. Penn helped with the chapters on retirement planning.

Sue Wollenweber, Cathy Capron, Bernadette Denoyer, and Linda Brzezinski helped with the last minute rush to pull the chapters together.

I appreciate the patience of the other financial and investment planners in my firm, Barry A. Riske, Jerry R. Jenkins, Jeff K. Pashe, and Dennis J. Prout while the staff set their work aside to get this book out on time. I also appreciate their support during the writing of *Financial Strategies for Physicians*.

Most of all, I would like to thank my clients who have given me their trust and loyalty and confidence, which made *Financial Strategies for Physicians* a reality.

Contents

Preface

In the past, and even today, many physicians achieved financial success in spite of themselves. Physician's incomes were very high. Even after inflation and taxes, physicians had great amounts of discretionary cash to set aside to assure financial well-being.

Yet many physicians did not do this and today they are feeling the effects of taxation, inflation, and competition, all of which are affecting their income, lifestyle, and financial well-being.

In 1970 there was 1 physician for every 658 Americans. By 1983 the ration was 1 for every 485 Americans. According to the Graduate Medical Education Advisory Committee (GMEAC) the ideal ratio is 1 M.D. for every 524 Americans. In fact, the GMEAC predicts by 1990 there will be 70,000 more M.D.s than needed.

The financially successful physicians of the future are going to be the physicians who arrange their practice and financial affairs with a practical businessperson's approach. This book is designed for those people who want to attain and maintain financial well-being. Financial well-being does not mean having $1,000,000. in your pension plan, or an adequate life insurance program. It means having your financial affairs arranged in such a way as to assure the attainment of your immediate, intermediate, and long range goals. Financial planning is a "process" of arranging your assets and income to achieve financial well-being. Financial planning is more quantitative while financial well-being is qualitative.

Chances are you picked up this book because you are feeling financially frustrated or have this nagging feeling that, perhaps, you are not running your financial affairs so as to assure your money is being utilized to maximum efficiency. Perhaps you are feeling overwhelmed by all the financial data thrown at you by insurance agents, securities brokers, banks, trust companies, financial planners, colleagues, spouses, and best friends. Perhaps you feel as if you have walked into the House of 31 Flavors only to find out they are out of your first, second, and third choices.

It is not going to get better; making financial choices and decisions will be harder as our system becomes more complex. However, choices have to be made and financial choices are much harder to make than deciding upon an ice cream cone. This book will help making those choices easier by helping you separate essential data from nonessential.

Financial Strategies for Physicians is written for those individuals willing to take responsibility to achieve financial well-being. To attain financial well-being, you must deal with reality. You must take the blinders off, to see where you are financially.

There are 14 primary goals I wish to achieve in writing this book:

1. Help you increase your productivity and potential of your practice to leave you more bottom-line $$'s.
2. Help you analyze where you are today and help you make concrete your goals and objectives.
3. Help explain how you can develop a strategy to attain your financial goals and to give you the specific tools with which to attain those goals and objectives.
4. Illustrate those specific strategies that can be operationalized to assure the attainment of your goals, such as, what type of investment program is best for you, how to use your business to increase your wealth-building ability, etc.
5. Describe how to use 100 percent no-risk (*Financial Strategies for Physicians* will teach you that all investments have risk) strategies to create wealth for yourself at maximum efficiency.
6. How to educate your children without going broke.
7. How to invest your money so that it grows and why you should have only one investment goal.
8. Identify the specific investment strategies you should utilize and how your portfolio should be managed.
9. Describe how to retire rich and what retirement is.
10. Describe how you should structure your estate to assure your family's security.
11. Explain why Uncle Sam can make you rich and how to make the "tax laws" your friend.
12. Give you some samples of other financial plans that you can use to help you design your own financial plan based on your own quantitative and qualitative needs (planning by values).
13. Describe how to develop a financial plan of action that pulls together all the financial strategies and tools outlined in this book.
14. Explain how to use financial planning professionals to implement certain financial strategies. Show you how to use your experts and what to expect and not expect from your advisors.

You get nothing for nothing out of life. To achieve financial well-being requires investment of your time to learn about how money works. This book will give you the tools to build financial well-being; however, it is up to you to make your "declaration of financial independence."

There is an old Mid-eastern proverb that reads, "Blessed is the man that gives advice, but 1,000 times more blessed is the man who takes that advice, and uses it."

Read on. . . .

Learn what you have to gain.

1

Your Most Important Investment—Yourself

As a physician, the first place you should invest your money and time is in increasing your practice's profit potential (in other words, you.) If you plan on going into practice for yourself, then you must look at yourself as a mini-conglomerate, whose skills must be marketed efficiently and whose major capital expense is the outlay you expended to educate yourself.

You (physician/businessperson) should market your practice in order to increase its potential profits and income. If you wish to be employed by someone else, either through a group practice or hospital, you should consider yourself similar to a major league athlete whose skills go to the highest bidder.

If you choose to work at a group practice or for a large medical corporation or hospital, naturally you should evaluate the workstyle that you desire, but, very importantly, you must also consider all the cash benefit compensation that will be paid to you for your skills. Your skills should be marketed effectively and efficiently to allow you to achieve whatever financial goals you may have.

This chapter will deal with the methods for you to increase your ability to produce a favorable income for yourself and your family. Many physicians do not like to look at themselves as self-employed. They prefer to perceive themselves as and orient their careers toward working for a major corporation or someone else in a group practice.

It is very important to understand that everyone is self-employed, and we get paid according to our ability to market ourselves, utilize our skills, and fill the need for our services. Many physicians may argue that they like the security of working for a big corporation. However, there is no security in working for someone else, since businesses fail each day and your corporate career can be as precarious as the whims of the personnel director or the chief staff physician.

If you choose to work for someone else, you should have an employment contract with that company, spelling out exactly what your duties and obligations to the company are, your cash compensation, fringe benefits, whether they will pay for your malpractice insurance, how you could be fired, and the consequences of quitting, becoming disabled, retiring, etc.

Many physicians who go to work in a practice do not like the cold regimentation of having an employment contract and feel that it is a slap in the face to their employer to ask for one. They liken it to a premarriage agreement, where you start planning for divorce before you are even married. Our careers are not like marriages, however, and they should be treated as a business.

If your potential employer will not consent to an employment agreement, then the decision is up to you as to whether you want to work without contract, knowing you could be fired a few days before you vest for that retirement plan, or as soon as the son of the senior person in practice graduates from medical school.

Following are some of the very important points that you should have in your employment agreement:

1. What will be my salary
2. Will I participate in my fees? When? How much?
3. What will you expect me to generate in fees (1st year, 2nd year) from working for you?
4. How many days of paid vacation do I get?
5. What holidays do I get?
6. Who pays for continuing education credits?
7. What if I get sick or die?
8. What type of retirement plan?
9. How can I be fired?
10. Is moonlighting O.K.?
11. Who pays for health insurance?
12. Is my disability benefit insured or a promise of the corporation?
13. What do I get if I quit?
14. What will it cost to buy into this practice?
15. Who pays malpractice?

Whenever you go to work for someone else, you should sit down with your potential employer and go over what is expected of you so that everything is spelled out and understood, regardless of whether you are going to have an employment contract or not. The questions in the above list should be considered and discussed in detail with your employer before you go to work.

THE PHYSICIAN/BUSINESSPERSON

You as a physician/businessperson must manage your practice like a business. You must market your skills in a cost-effective efficient manner. If you are a physician starting your career you will find a horrendous amount of competition for patients and medical care and you must establish yourself in business quickly to generate a cash flow to support your business and your personal lifestyle income needs.

For those physicians who have been in practice for quite some time, you must be able to maintain the share of the market that you gained over the years and have your patient load increase in order to offset that which you will lose because of death, retirement, moving to another part of the country, or those that go to competitors.

A physician is in a service business and the client relationship is generally ongoing. You trade your skills for your patients' money. The best marketing plan is to have your clients feel like you really care about their well being and that you serve their needs in a cost-effective pleasant manner. As a physician/businessperson you should examine very carefully the procedures you use for patient care, including the way your staff works with your patients and other physicians, all of whom are potential referral sources. If you feel you have developed these areas to where new patients are being treated as they want to be treated, then you must consider ways and methodologies to increase your patient flow consistent with the character of professionalism.

When most physicians do an analysis of where they get most of their patients, they will find that the majority of their patients come from referrals. As a general practitioner, you will find that referrals come from patients who are satisfied and very happy with you, and thus, refer their friends and acquaintances. For the physician who specializes, you will also find that a large portion of patients come from referrals, whether from the hospital, other physicians, or former patients. Thus, you must look at everyone you come into contact with, especially your patients and the other professionals with whom you work, as your marketing force. You must look at them as your practice's salespeople as they are going to go out and tell others about your services, whether good or bad. If you treated your patient or other physicians (potential referrers) rudely, then you can expect them to go out and market the fact that you are brusque, egotistical, rude, and not a very pleasant person.

If your salespeople go out telling how pleasant you are, and about your wonderful staff, and how you took the time to explain to your patient their problem so they felt like a person and not a number, then you can expect that person to go out and tell friends, relatives, and acquaintances, and these people are naturally going to gravitate towards your practice.

Figure 1-1 is a sample practice ethics statement that you should go over with each of your employees, naturally modifying it to your own values.

If you are a specialist and your manner is brusque and you treat the staff at the hospital in a rude and "holier than thou" manner, you could expect that the referrals they have for your specialty are going to go to your competitor who treats colleagues and support staff with kindness and respect.

Naturally for the physician who is just starting out in practice, it takes a while before people find out what a wonderful person you are, and in order to help generate patients, there are a few simple steps to follow to help increase patient flow:

1. Send out press releases to the local media about your background an-
   nouncing that you are setting up practice in the local community. In
   addition to this, placing advertisements for a few weeks in the local
   publications indicating that you are new in business and taking new
   patients, can be very helpful.
2. Putting on Continuing Education classes pertaining to your specialty at
   the local community college can help bring in patients, with seminar
   topics that are similar to your specialty. If you are a general practitioner,
   seminars about nutrition, pre and post natal care, birthing, sports
   medicine, etc., can all be very helpful.

For the specialist whose practice will depend heavily on the referrals of
other physicians, maintaining a high profile by writing in professional
journals and by taking other physicians out to breakfast or lunch, etc., can
be very helpful. Figure 1-2 is a chart of how physicians plan and promote
their practices. Figure 1-3 is a market research worksheet that should be
helpful in evaluating your specific market. Both you and a staff member
should complete the form, and you should discuss your answers to this
worksheet with your staff and use it in promoting your practice.

Corporate Goal:
Provide our clients with high-quality health care that helps assure clients'
wellbeing . . .
And provide positive, creative environment where self-managers can grow and
prosper to the mutual benefit of our clients and ourselves.

Practice Ethics:
1. Each employee shall be a "self-manager" working within a framework of
   "priorities."
2. Each self-manager will subscribe to the following ethics:
    • Honesty always
    • Accomplishment oriented
    • Client is always to be treated as if he/she was our only client
    • No hierarchy
    • 100% total confidentiality
    • "Get it done right the first time" orientation
    • Proper dress, hygiene, and manners
    • Commitment to lifelong education to keep skills sharp and assure that
      we stay on the vanguard
    • Re-inventor of the company and the procedures by making suggestions
      (and implementing them) that will make the company and yourself
      more efficient and profitable
    • Adherence to the Golden Rule

Fig. 1-1. Sample practice ethics statement.

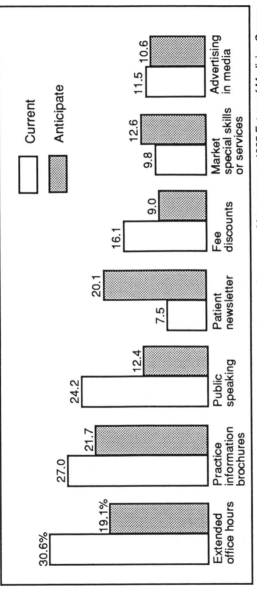

FUTURE OF MEDICINE SURVEY
HOW WILL PHYSICIANS BE PROMOTING THEIR PRACTICES?

We asked the physicians in our survey sample what practice promotion techniques they are currently using and what techniques they anticipate using within the next 5 years.

Current

Anticipate

Extended office hours — 30.6% / 19.1%

Practice information brochures — 27.0 / 21.7

Public speaking — 24.2 / 12.4

Patient newsletter — 7.5 / 20.1

Fee discounts — 16.1 / 9.0

Market special skills or services — 9.8 / 12.6

Advertising in media — 11.5 / 10.6

Total exceeds 100% due to multiple responses.
N=653 (100% of survey sample)

Source: PHYSICIAN's MANAGEMENT's *1985 Future of Medicine Survey.*
Copyright © 1985 by Harcourt Brace Jovanovich, Inc. All rights reserved.

Fig. 1-2. Future of medicine survey. How will physicians be promoting their practices? Physicians in the survey sample what practice promotion techniques they are currently using and what techniques they anticipate using within the next 5 years. From Physician's Management's *1985 Future of Medicine Survey.* Orlando, Harcourt Brace Jovanovich, Inc. With permission.

MARKET RESEARCH—WORKSHEET

A. Brief statement of medical practice you are in.

B. Specific definition of your services.

C. What percentage of your patients are: Self-referred _____

Physician referred _____ Hospital referred _____

D. List and rank reasons why physicians refer to you.

                                                                    Rank

1. _____   _____

2. _____   _____

3. _____   _____

E. List and rank three common characteristics of your referring
physicians.

                                                                    Rank

1. _____   _____

2. _____   _____

3. _____   _____

F. List and rank reasons why patients use your services.

                                                                    Rank

1. _____   _____

2. _____   _____

3. _____   _____

G. List and rank three common characteristics of your patients.

                                                                    Rank

1. _____   _____

2. _____   _____

3. _____   _____

H. Referral Profile:

1. Number of total patients in market area _____

2. Number of total physicians in market area _____

3. Number of total hospitals in market area _____

Fig. 1-3. Market research worksheet. (From Mary Bevans Gillett, Marketing Communicatons Consultant, Traverse City, MI 49684. With permission.)

MARKET RESEARCH—WORKSHEET

I. Fill in the blanks for a typical patient.

    a. Where located _____

    b. Male _____   Female _____

    c. Age range _____

    d. Income bracket _____

    e. Occupation _____

    f. Education level _____

    g. _____   _____

    h. _____   _____

J. List the main competition in your market area. Estimate annual practice income and percent of the total market.

Competitor	Estimated Income	Percent Total
_____	_____	_____
_____	_____	_____
_____	_____	_____

K. Rate your competition—overall in market area.

Strengths	Weaknesses
_____	_____
_____	_____
_____	_____

L. Advantages of my practice over competition.

Services _____

Location _____

Hospital affiliation _____

Availability _____

Office Staff _____

Fees/Billing Practices _____

Professional Training _____

Office Practices _____

As a family practitioner, hiring older, experienced staff can be very helpful as often these people have a high profile in the community and can thus work to help bring in a very steady patient load through their former acquaintances and patients. Also, contacting the local life insurance agencies stating that you do insurance medical exams, can make a difference.

Talk shows on radio and television can be very helpful as can an "Ask Dr. Jones" weekly editorial in the local newspaper. As you build your practice to a size you are happy with, it is very important that you continually look at making sure you are spending your money in a prudent cost-effective manner, to increase your practice's profit potential. You should place yourself near where you want your patients to come from. If you are a specialist, then you should try to be near your hospital so that you don't have to spend a lot of time traveling. Your staff should be lean, your billing procedure efficient, orderly, and consistent.

You should talk to other physicians if you are opening a practice, and learn from them on how to set up your practice. Many physicians ask their medical suppliers how to set up their practices and that is sort of asking the wolf to guard the henhouse. Ask your physician colleagues, accountant, attorney, or financial planning professionals who specialize in working with physicians how to set up your office in a cost-effective manner.

Since staff salaries are one of the biggest budgetary expenses that you will have, you should only hire a new staff person after everyone in your office, including yourself, is feeling the stress of overwork. Then, and only then, should a new staff person be hired, to fill the void and to take the tremendous workload off the other staff people. If you start out with a large staff and a modest amount of work, the employer's rule is, the employee's work will expand to fill the time allotted for the task.

The bottom line for the physicians of the future will be that you must run your practice like a business and you must control costs since the competition for patients is going to become fierce in the future.

As mentioned in this book's introduction, the Graduate Medical Education Advisory Committee estimates that by 1990 there will be 70,000 more M.D.s than are needed, and to be financially successful as a physician in the future, you are going to have to manage your practice in a practical, cost-effective, intelligent, and prudent manner.

Appendices A-D should be read and used by you to help in advertising and promoting your practices to assure long-term financial success.

RECOMMENDED READING

Hill N: Laws of Success. Success Unlimited, Inc., Chicago, IL, 1979

McCormack MH: What They Don't Teach You at Harvard Business School. Notes from a Street Smart Executive, INC Magazine, Bantam Books, New York, N.Y. 1985. In Search of Excellence—Laws of Success

Peters J and Waterman H, Jr: In Search of Excellence—Lessons from America's Best Run Companies, Harper Row, New York, N.Y., 1982

Appendix A
PUBLIC RELATION TIPS

Every business has public relations; the PR may be good, bad, or in between. A good PR program starts with the owners of the business and permeates the organization in good employee relations as well as good company relations with the outside world.

Use the following simple rules as a guide to good public relations.

1. Work actively at getting as much PR as you can.
2. Submit all newsworthy events about your business.
3. Learn and use news release style and format.
4. Try not to con the press or media.
5. Be available to the media for comment. Be aware of news deadlines.
6. Avoid misunderstanding and misquotes by translating scientific and medical terminology into easily understood examples.
7. Always issue counter-statements to negative press.
8. Don't forget the trade and industry publications.
9. Develop mailing lists of trade publications, general community publications, community leaders, competitors and customers.
10. Consider publishing a patient and/or referring physician newsletter.
11. Establish relations and build rapport with media, community, etc.
12. Keep files: general information; your releases and articles; your competitors' releases and articles.
13. An upset customer is bad PR.
14. Good service is good PR.

Source: Mary Bevans Gillett, Marketing Communications Consultant, Traverse City, MI 49684. With permission.

Appendix B
ADVERTISING TIPS

The following are some general tips for developing and evaluating your advertising.

1. Maintain consistency. Once you've defined your image, select your logo, look and sound to achieve it. Includes style consistency in typeface, graphics/layout, audio/music, photography, illustrations, format, etc. Consistency reinforces your image and helps your customers recognize your ads immediately.
2. Advertise products or services that have merit in themselves. Unless a product or service is good, few customers will make a repeat purchase . . . regardless of advertising.
3. Know exactly what you wish a particular ad to accomplish. In an immediate response ad, you want customers to come in and buy items in the next several days. In attitude advertising, you are creating and maintaining long-term image and awareness.
4. Plan the ad around one idea. Each ad should only have one message. If that needs reinforcement with other ideas, keep them in the background. If you have several important things to say, use a different ad for each one and run them on succeeding days or weeks.
5. Identify your business fully and clearly. Logos should be clean lined, uncluttered and prominently displayed. Hours, telephone number, directions, similar appropriate information should also be included.
6. Treat messages seriously. Humor is risky and difficult to write. Be creative but be on the safe side. Tell people the facts about the merchandise or services.
7. Make copy simple. Write the message conversationally and try to get the point across in the first sentence.
8. Use direct, persuasive wording. Don't use worn out cliches, think of a unique saying to fit your special circumstances.
9. Show the benefit to the reader. Give the customer one primary reason to buy, then mention one or two secondary reasons.
10. Show your product/service in use, what it looks like, the result of its use, etc. With radio, paint a visual image through words and sound effects.
11. Assess the advertising climate in your medical community. Plan campaign accordingly.

Source: Mary Bevans Gillett, Marketing Communications Consultant, Traverse City, MI 49684. With permission.

Appendix C
MARKETING COMMUNICATIONS "SHOPPING LIST"

Every piece of written, printed, electronic and verbal material can be considered "Marketing Communications." The following lists examples in the main categories of general business communications, public relations and advertising.

General Business Communications

General and promotional information about your firm as well as printed materials needed for day-to-day operation. Includes:

LOGO	A-V PRESENTATIONS (informational)
BUSINESS CARDS	STOREFRONT/SIGN
LETTERHEAD	PATIENT EDUCATION MATERIAL
INVOICES	3RD PARTY PAYER INFORMATION
SALES RECEIPTS	FOLDERS
PRACTICE BROCHURE	

Public Relations

Often referred to as "free advertising," PR is basically the eyes, ears and mouth of your organization. Purpose is to promote goodwill and enhance company image. Includes:

NEWS RELEASES	MEDIA RELATIONS
RADIO/TV PSAs	COMMUNITY INVOLVEMENT
SEMINARS/WORKSHOPS	SPECIAL EVENTS/PROMOTIONS
CME TALKS	HEALTH FAIR

Advertising

Paid communication whose purpose is to "impart information, develop attitudes and induce favorable action for the advertiser." Includes:

DIRECT MAIL	DISPLAY ADS (PRINT MEDIA)
POSTERS—INFORMATIONAL	COMMERCIALS (ELECTRONIC MEDIA)
DISPLAYS—INFORMATIONAL	YELLOW PAGES/DIRECTORIES
SPECIALTY ADVERTISING	TRADE PUBLICATIONS/MAGAZINES

Remember, this is only a sampling of the numerous marketing communication options available. Your marketing strategy should incorporate the promotional vehicles needed to meet your goals based on your market research, your budget and your three-year plan.

Source: Mary Bevans Gillett, Marketing Communications Consultant, Traverse City, MI 49684. With permission.

Appendix D
ADDITIONAL GENERAL TIPS ON PHYSICIAN MARKETING

1. *Review your office practices.* Are you usually on schedule? Are long patient waiting times the exception or the rule? Does your office staff explain when you are delayed and offer to reschedule patients?
2. *Practice "guest relations."* Guest relations is simply common courtesy. Is your office staff friendly, courteous and helpful? Your receptionist is usually the first line of communication between you and your patient. Rudeness and inefficiency, via the phone or in person, reflects poorly on your practice.
3. *Provide patient education materials.* Have general information (i.e., brochures, magazines, etc.) available in your waiting areas. Provide specific disease or procedure information to patients as needed. Use anatomical models. Recommend further reading, information sources or support groups. Translate medical jargon into everyday language. Consider publishing a patient newsletter.
4. *Communicate.* Greet your patients in a friendly, relaxed manner. Remember that many people, especially the elderly, resent being addressed by their first name. Actively listen to what your patients are saying. Answer your patients' questions as directly as possible, avoiding jargon and explaining in easily understood terms. Encourage patients to ask questions and learn more about their condition. Explain your method of treatment, alternatives, recovery, etc. Offer to discuss treatment or illness with a spouse or family member. Ask questions to ascertain your patients' understanding of diagnosis and general health principles.
5. *Communicate billing policies.* Discuss your fees and billing policies in advance so payment will not become a negative issue later. Make sure office staff is familiar with third party regulations, hospital billing procedures, etc. and can help assist patients.
6. *Consider altering schedule or office set-up to address patient needs.* If many of your patients work from 9–5, consider periodically offering Saturday morning or early morning hours. Have a small table, coloring books and a few children's toys available for young patients or siblings. Consider a satellite clinic in rural areas.
7. *Interface with colleagues, administrators and referring physicians.* Be actively involved in medical staff practices and decisions. Participate in CME courses and medical seminars. Offer to speak on your specialty and keep up to date with advances in other fields.
8. *Communicate with referring physicians.* Keep referring physicians aware of their patients' status. Follow-up with phone calls, letters and operative and discharge summaries. Keep lines of communication open.
9. *Remember that "marketing" is not just selling or advertising.* We are in a competitive environment. However, marketing begins in the office and

at the bedside . . . communicating with patients, responding to their needs and providing high quality health care. A flashy ad campaign will never compensate for poor medical treatment, sloppy office practices or a rude staff.

Source: Mary Bevans Gillett, Marketing Communications Consultant, Traverse City, MI 49684. With permission.

Give Yourself a Financial Exam

2

The starting block for developing a financial strategy is to find out where you are and where you want to be. The inability to set financial goals and priorities and to take action on those goals and priorities is the number 1 reason that people fail financially. For physicians, taking the time to decide on goals and priorities is often put on the back burner because of the demands and pressures that are imposed on physicians by themselves, clients, society, a hectic work environment, and their family.

To set goals and objectives, it is important that you divorce yourself from analyzing beyond the goals. For example, don't say, "There's nothing I can do about my debt or the amount of money I'm paying in taxes."

Write down as a goal, "I want to get my debt structure and budget under control." Set a goal of "My goal is to reduce taxes, so that I have more money to spend where I wish it to be spent." We find that most physicians have the following goals:

1. Reduce taxes (all physicians who pay taxes should have this goal).
2. Have a properly structured debt situation.
3. Have an efficient practice.
4. Create wealth for children's education, financial security, retirement, to allow the physician to slow down as they mature, etc.
5. To arrange affairs so as to minimize the impact of death to their families.
6. To maximize the performance of their investments.
7. To arrange their affairs so they can slow down and have a shorter work week resulting in less stress, better quality of life, etc.

The primary goal that seems to come up in the dozens of interviews I've had with physician/clients is that they are searching for financial direction that encompasses all of the above goals and objectives, and is consistent with their value system. A financial plan should reflect a person's value system.

Dale Edwin grew up in a small farming town outside of metropolitan Detroit area. His father was a low-paid night watchman for a utility company and the family got by growing much of their food on their small farm and by selling butter and eggs to neighbors. Dale and his four brothers helped with the farm and worked hard to complete high school. Dale wanted more for himself than being a night watchman and on graduation from high school, Dale wrestled his way into college. He worked his way through college by waitering, lifeguarding in Florida during the spring breaks, washing dishes, and helping out at the Y.M.C.A.

In 1952 he married a graduate from Ohio State University. Dale's wife already had her degree and taught nursery school and swimming to help put him through school. A few years later, just after Dale got his undergraduate degree, a child was born and Dale was forced to take a full-time job. He still wanted to be a physician and continued to pursue his degree. Finally in 1956 he achieved his goal and set up a practice in pediatrics. By now there were two children and another on the way. Dale set about opening up his practice that, because of his down to earth nature, became very successful. Naturally there were a few rough spots in the first few years but luckily his wife was able to bring in that second income to help support the family.

Dale and his wife decided before Dale went into practice that he would never work beyond 4:00 P.M. weekdays, take weekends off, and in the summers have a four-day practice. He spent his evenings with his family going to the ball games, hiking, swimming, and fishing for coho salmon out in front of their Lake Michigan home.

Dale's earnings from his practice never got above $40,000–$50,000 a year. He always said that if he would start earning more money than that he would take more time off, because spending time with his family was more important than making more money. Every year he would set aside a small percentage of his income toward retirement and he told his children he would try to help them with college, but that they should start developing their skills so that they could put themselves through college as he had.

He taught his children as he had lived, that life was a long time and they, without having a lot of anxiety, could leisurely go about accomplishing their goals. Dale never talked about retirement except to say that "I'm already retired because I'm living exactly the way I want to live, today."

Dale died at age 53, with 4 children at home aged 14–18. This was a few years ago and I've talked to the children. None of them feel that Dale missed out on life and they all admired him for his ability to live a balanced life. They all joked that Dale never bought a new car and that the boat they went fishing in cost $200, and they laughed as they explained that the engine used to always konk out in the middle of Lake Michigan.

Dale had lived his value system and it was reflected in the way he ran his finances. His finances revolved around his lifestyle. He made sure his insurance program was adequate so that his family was taken care of should he die or get disabled. He said that the best thing that he could give his family was himself and from talking to his six children, they all agree.

Dale Apple, on the other hand, had one goal, and that was to retire at age 50 with $1,000,000. Dr. Apple took the few extra years of school to become a surgeon and set up a practice that became very successful. His earnings were in the $300,000–$400,000 range annually. He'd put as much money as he could into tax shelters, his retirement plans, and other investments. He worked 5–6 days a week and went to seminars to sharpen his skills on weekends and his time off. When people would ask him why he worked so hard, he'd say that at age 50 he was hanging up his scalpel.

Dr. Apple died of a stroke at age 44. His first, second, and third wives and their four children attended the funeral. Dr. Apple had a substantial amount of money set aside toward achieving his goal of retiring at age 50. Not as much as he had hoped to, however, as child support and alimony payments had eaten up a substantial amount of the money he had planned to set aside for retirement.

When you ask Apple's children about their father, they all bring up the week he couldn't work because he slipped in the bath tub and sprained his hand. Dr. Apple, unable to do surgery, took his kids to Disneyland. They joke about it, and when you look into their eyes you wonder if they greased the tub.

Financial planning is a process whereby you allocate your assets and your income to meet your goals. Your goals are affected by your value system. Most people's value systems fall somewhere between Dr. Edwin's and Dr. Apple's.

Figure 2-1 is a flow chart to help you better understand the chronology of setting up a financial plan for yourself. Below are some questions you should ask yourself to help you get a better "feel" for your goals and objectives and your value system.

LIFESTYLE QUESTIONS

How many days a week do I want to spend in practice? Do I want to take a vacation every year, and how much time do I want to take off for that vacation? Am I happy with the structure of my practice, or should I bring in a partner, go out on my own, or go into a corporate practice?

Figure 2-2 is a financial statement that should be filled out so that you can get an idea of where you are today, financially. This chapter is not going to deal with the specifics of risk management or wealth accumulation; however, it is very important that you ask yourself the Lifestyle Questions (above) so you are able to prioritize your situation first.

The cornerstone of a financial plan is to make sure your insurance program is adequate and efficient. A physician is a money machine. The physician's skills produce income and the average income of physicians is around $95,000 a year. If you had a machine that had the potential to produce $95,000 a year, you would surely insure that machine's ability to continue to produce a substantial income. Proper disability, life, and health insurance are extremely important and should not be considered investments but, rather, should be considered as the cost of doing business. Casualty coverage should be reviewed periodically, as should other types of coverage such as malpractice insurance and other liability insurance. The chapter on risk management will deal with this in greater detail; however, you should ask yourself these questions:

- What lifestyle would I want if I become permanently disabled? How much income would I need to support that lifestyle?
- What lifestyle would I want for my family should I die? How much income would they need to support that lifestyle?
- Am I adequately protected against major catastrophe, no matter how remote?
- Regarding supporting lifestyle wealth accumulation goals, you should ask yourself:

HOW TO ALLOCATE YOUR ASSETS TO MEET YOUR GOALS

Proper financial planning involves the allocation of your assets and income to accomplish your financial and personal objectives.

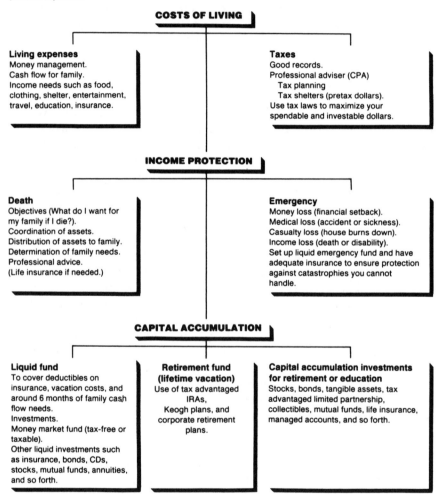

COSTS OF LIVING

Living expenses
Money management.
Cash flow for family.
Income needs such as food,
clothing, shelter, entertainment,
travel, education, insurance.

Taxes
Good records.
Professional adviser (CPA)
   Tax planning
   Tax shelters (pretax dollars).
Use tax laws to maximize your
   spendable and investable dollars.

INCOME PROTECTION

Death
Objectives (What do I want for
my family if I die?).
Coordination of assets.
Distribution of assets to family.
Determination of family needs.
Professional advice.
(Life insurance if needed.)

Emergency
Money loss (financial setback).
Medical loss (accident or sickness).
Casualty loss (house burns down).
Income loss (death or disability).
Set up liquid emergency fund and have
adequate insurance to ensure protection
against catastrophies you cannot
handle.

CAPITAL ACCUMULATION

Liquid fund
To cover deductibles on
insurance, vacation costs, and
around 6 months of family cash
flow needs.
Investments.
Money market fund (tax-free or
taxable).
Other liquid investments such
as insurance, bonds, CDs,
stocks, mutual funds, annuities,
and so forth.

**Retirement fund
(lifetime vacation)**
Use of tax advantaged
IRAs,
Keogh plans, and
corporate retirement
plans.

**Capital accumulation investments
for retirement or education**
Stocks, bonds, tangible assets, tax
advantaged limited partnership,
collectibles, mutual funds, life insurance,
managed accounts, and so forth.

Note: This chart should not be considered legal or accounting advice. Seek competent professional help to assist you in
       accomplishing your financial goals.

Fig. 2-1.

© **FINANCIAL & INVESTMENT MANAGEMENT GROUP**
PENSION SERVICE DESIGN, INC./FINANCIAL & INVESTMENT PLANNING LTD

Date _____/_____/_____

Name_____

Social Sec. #'s _____/_____

Date (s) of Birth _____/_____

Children:

Name(s)	DOB	Name(s)	DOB
_____	___	_____	___
_____	___	_____	___

Business Phone# _____

Personal Phone# _____

Business Address _____

_____

Home Address_____

_____

Investment Assets

Cash/Checking & Money Fund(s) $ _____

Individual Retirement Account(s) _____

Retirement Plans . . . . _____

Limited Parnerships

(list separately) . . . . _____

Real Estate . . . . _____

. . . . _____

. . . . _____

Securities total

(list separately) . . . . _____

Lifestyle Assets

Personal Residence . . . . _____

Furniture/Appliances . . . . _____

Automobile(s) . . . . _____

Personal/Jewelry, art, etc. . . . . _____

. . . . _____

. . . . _____

Business Assets

Real Business Assets . . . . _____

Goodwill Value . . . . _____

. . . . _____

Total Assets . . . . $ _____

Income:

198__ Earned $_____
        Unearned $_____
        Total $_____

198__ Earned $_____
        Unearned $_____
        Total $_____

Present Year Esiimate:
Earned $_____
Unearned $_____
Total $_____

Liabilities

Home Mortgage (Pymt. $_____) $ _____

Balloon Year_____ Interest _____

Other Real Estate (Pymt. $_____) _____

Auto(s) (Pymt. $_____) (_____%)_____

(Pymt. $_____) (_____%)_____

. . . . _____

Notes Payable: (Pymt. $_____)
(Purpose _____) _____

Balloon Year_____ Interest_____

. . . . _____

Total Liabilities_____ $ _____

NET WORTH . . . . $ _____

Expenses

Fed. & State Income Taxes . . . . . . _____

Real Estate Taxes . . . . _____

Investment Accounts . . . . _____

Other Fixed Expenses . . . . _____

. . . . _____

. . . . _____

. . . . _____

Total . . . . $ _____

PERSONAL ADVISORS:

Accountant _____Phone#_____

Address _____

Attorney _____Phone#_____

Address _____

Bank & Officer_____

Casualty Agent _____Phone#_____

Fig. 2-2.

- ◆ Do I wish to educate my children? Do I wish to pay for pre-college, undergraduate, postgraduate?
- ◆ Is retirement important to me? (Our definition of retirement is "Working when you want, if you want, how you want and where you want.")
- ◆ What type of lifestyle do I want at retirement?
- ◆ How can I reduce taxes and have more money to spend now and in the future?
- ◆ Do I want major lifestyle-oriented properties such as a vacation home, boat, airplane, etc.?
- ◆ Is it important to me to build my net worth?
- Naturally everybody wants to reduce taxes and every legal means of reducing taxes should be taken to help create wealth for yourself, or to provide the freedom to do other things with that income.

Once you have set these goals you should prioritize them. Naturally, realistic balance is the key. For example, something will have to give if you want to retire a millionaire in 10 years, and only work 2 days a week. Reaching a proper balance is attainable and this will be discussed further in later chapters.

Figure 2-3 shows the forms we use in our practice to help a client get an idea of where they are financially—their goals, objectives, and priorities. None of these forms should be filled out until you have finished this book so that they are filled out with knowledge and understanding of the financial principles that will help you achieve your financial goals. If you are married, it would be helpful to have your spouses also read this book so that their input is considered, as you develop your own personal strategies for financial success.

INCOME & TAX PLANNING

Is your income predictable? Yes_____ No_____

Do you plan on changing your present work position in the future? Yes_____ No_____

Do you have a line of credit? Yes_____ No_____ Amount_____Financial Institution Name .

Have you ever done any income tax planning? Yes_____ No_____ If yes, please explain.

_____

TAX PLANNING VEHICLES (Please submit pertinent documents.)

_____IRA   _____Deferred Compensation Plan _____Tax Sheltered Custodial A/C

_____Retirement trust   _____Limited Parnerships   _____Others (Please list)

_____Interest Free Loans _____501(c)9 V.E.B.A. Trusts   _____

ADDITIONAL BENEFITS. (Please submit the pertinent documents.)

_____Salary Continuation Plan   _____Interest Free Loans

_____Sick Pay/Disability   _____Company Car

_____Health Insurance   _____Dues/Memberships

_____Medical Reimbursement Plan   _____Others (Please list)_____

_____Group Life Insurance   _____

If incorporated, date of incorporation: _____/_____/_____

Type of Corporation (P.C., Regular, or "Sub S")_____

FINANCIAL INDEPENDENCE INFORMATION

How much money do you estimate you need per month to provide for your basic living expenses (food, clothing, housing, entertainment, travel, etc.)? $_____

At what age do you wish to retire?_____

What do you feel that your investment assets should do for you? _____

_____

In terms of your assets directed to investment areas, please rate how you feel about the following statements:

	Strongly Agree	Agree	Disagree	No Opinion
A. Short term safety of capital is very important				
B. Longer term safety of capital is very important				
C. Inflation protection (maintenance of purchasing power) is very important				
D. I am interested in pursuing **growth Investments** and I'm willing to take the higher risks involved				
E. Income is very important to me				
F. A balanced program of income and growth investments makes the most sense to someone in my circumstances				
G. The idea of a professional manager assisting me in managing my investments to capitalize on opportunities and reduce risks through active management makes sense to me				

Fig. 2-3A.

©FINANCIAL & INVESTMENT MANAGEMENT GROUP
PENSION SERVICE DESIGN, INC./FINANCIAL & INVESTMENT PLANNING LTD

I understand the cyclical nature of longer term investments. Yes_____ No_____

CHILDREN'S EDUCATION

Have you considered setting aside money for your children's education? Yes_____ No_____

If yes, which levels of their education would you be paying for: Pre-college Yes_____ No_____

Undergraduate Yes_____ No_____, Post-graduate Yes_____ No_____.

What percentage of your children's education do you feel should be paid for by the child through government loans, summer work, etc.? _____%

Do you visualize any changes in your lifestyle upon your retirement? Yes_____ No_____

If yes, please explain_____

_____

In "today's dollars", how much after-tax monthly income do you feel you will need upon retirement. $_____.

FINANCIAL SECURITY NEEDS

What does financial security mean to you?_____

_____

If you were to become disabled before retirement, how much monthly after-tax income would you need to maintain a comfortable standard of living? $_____

Are there any unusual medical histories or financial circumstances that should be discussed regarding you or your dependents? _____

_____

How much money would you want in a highly liquid state such as a savings account for an emergency or opportunity reserve? $_____

Do you have Wills or related Trust Agreements? Yes_____ No_____ If yes, when was the last time they were reviewed?_____

	PRIORITIES		
	TOP PRIORITY	PRIORITY	TO BE CONSIDERED
To reduce my personal income taxes			
To accumulate sufficient assets to provide an adequate after-tax retirement income.			
To provide for my children's education			
To provide a monthly after-tax income of $_____ for my family in the event I become ill or disabled.			
To build my net worth			
To arrange my affairs to minimize the impact of my death on my family			
To maximize the performance of my investment asset			
Other: _____			

_____
_____

Fig. 2-3B.

3
What is Financial Success?

Financial success is different for everybody. In Chapter 2 you filled out forms stating your objectives regarding your finances, investments, and insurance programs. These goals will reflect your value system; however, each goal must have a plan to achieve it, and each plan to achieve that goal will have a price that is paid, either in your time or with money. Gaining a balance between your personal, family, and practice goals can be very difficult. Making use of financial and investment tools and techniques will add "financial speed" to your goals. This financial speed, or efficiency, will allow you to spend more time with your family and pursuing personal lifestyle goals. This chapter will deal with the qualitative aspects of financial planning—where you set about attaining your goals in a relaxed and poised manner.

Dr. Jenkins, with 5 years in General Practice, who is married with 2 children, was feeling under pressure by decisions and choices he must make over the next year or so. Among these decisions were: (1) Consider bringing in a practicing associate. How would he compensate this person? Should he bring him or her in as a partner? How will his patients feel about not being able to deal directly with himself; (2) Should he limit his practice and not take on more patients, or would this be counter-productive since he may not be replacing the patients that he loses through attrition; (3) The local hospital has offered him a position running their sports medicine department and he finds this idea exciting and challenging and feels it would be very fulfilling for him. However, he feels an obligation to his existing patients, and his total income would be reduced from its current level if he took this new job. Now that he has two young children he wants to spend more time with them, but he is finding that he is getting home much later than he has in the past because his patients have grown accustomed to spending lots of time discussing their health care needs with him and because of emergencies and walk-in-patients who grew used to not having a regularly scheduled appointment.

Dr. Jenkins' wife, Julie, is constantly reminding him that when they were initially married they had decided that they would share in the raising of their children and the household duties. Dr. Jenkins wants to fulfill this commitment and the idea of spending time with his family is consistent with his value system. As he reminds Julie daily, however, the mortgage payment must be made and food must be put on the table. Making the transition to spending more time at home seems to be an impossibility right now because Dr. Jenkins hates to turn away business, finds his work fulfilling, and he needs the money.

In addition to the above mentioned stresses in Dr. Jenkins' life, last year, Dr. Jenkins' (who is an only child) widowed mother had a stroke and now will require full-time health care. Dr. Jenkins is feeling that he should make the arrangements for his mother, and is feeling pulled, frustrated, and out of control as he watches the people he loves and cares for drift slowly away from him.

Most people have not had to make the decisions that Dr. Jenkins will have to make in such a short time span. The stress of life, at times, can be very frustrating and a properly designed and executed financial plan can help reduce stress by anticipating events that will happen in a person's life and addressing them before they happen.

For example, in Dr. Jenkins' situation, if he knew that his financial situation was healthy, what his budget was, and what financial assets he has to help him achieve the type of lifestyle that he wants both now and in the future, he would be able to discuss with Julie and his patients whether or not he should go to work at the hospital. Thus, if Dr. Jenkins was on top of his financial life he would be able to isolate the financial aspects of working at the hospital and make it purely a lifestyle/workstyle decision.

Naturally, he will have to use many of the stress management techniques that he prescribes for his patients and he will start looking at his daily runs in light of stress management more than as a fun way of keeping fit.

As stated earlier, financial success is much different than financial well-being. Financial well-being helps anticipate problems and assures that assets are there so that finances do not add to the stresses in our life.

In Chapters 8–16, this book will discuss getting rich slowly and teach you how to have a balanced program to attain both financial success, and hopefully, assure financial well-being. This will allow you the freedom to live according to your own value system and to synthesize your value system with your goals and objectives.

To have a balanced lifestyle that fulfills you creatively, socially, and also makes you happy, in addition to achieving financial success, is a very hard task. While financial planning is arranging your assets and income to achieve your specific financial goals, financial success is the attainment of a feeling of well-being about your financial situation. A financially successful person is able to separate essential goals from nonessential goals, i.e., to make personal choices after analysis that make the most sense when considering your personal, family's, and colleagues' feelings. The financially successful person does not procrastinate and is able to make those difficult decisons. It is better to make a good decision now than to make an excellent decision in a month.

There is a buzz phrase in the financial community called "Planning by Objective." A person who is trying to increase the quality of his or her life, "plans by values." This person considers the family's feelings and goals and works with his or her spouse, colleagues, and children to formulate a plan that is fulfilling for oneself, family, and friends.

A major problem many physicians have is that they find that their work is extremely fulfilling and this allows them to hide in their work from family, social commitments, and self, all in the name of "financial security." If you find your work very fulfilling, then perhaps it makes more sense for you to consider working less hours, spending more time with your family at the expense of setting aside as much money toward retirement and planning on working a few more years past normal retirement, but having more balance today. An excellent book, *Looking Into The 21st Century*, mentions that there will be a trend toward people working shorter days, but into their 70s and 80s, not only for the reasons of economics, but because work is fun, fulfilling, and it gives purpose and meaning to our life. There is nothing wrong with getting rich slowly. Financial planning can help you get rich quick or slow. Your "financial speed" will depend on yourself and your own values.

Financial planning helps to achieve more quality by allowing you to have realistic goals that are thought out, and by keeping you from making big mistakes that could financially devastate you. Statisticians tells us that over half the divorces are caused by squabbles over money and most that do not fit in that category will say that the reason that the divorce came about was because they did not spend enough time working on their relationship.

Proper financial planning can help relieve the anxieties about money and make it so you can spend more time on your relationships. Achieving a proper balance between our personal lives and our business lives is one of the most difficult challenges we face today. However, you are in control of it. You are in control of your life.

4

Your Home and Other Real Estate

Physicians have real estate transactions for three specific reasons. They are: (1) housing (2) providing a work environment, and (3) investment.

While buying a home is an emotional decision, deciding on what type of office and where to locate your office should be considered strictly a business and financial decision. Reasons for purchasing real estate can cross over one another and you could have one property that acts as your office, home, and as an investment. Thus, you could find that one piece of real estate fulfills three good reasons to purchase one property. When purchasing a specific piece of real estate, however, it is important that you first analyze specifically why you are considering purchasing the property and what need you are fulfilling. This chapter will help you analyze your needs; deal with buying and selling your home; give you some specifics about your office and its location and on purchasing real estate for investment.

REAL ESTATE FOR HOUSING

Purchasing or renting real estate for housing should primarily be an emotional decision. Your home environment should make you feel comfortable, at ease, and relaxed. You should not make purchasing a home a financial decision, you should make it an emotional decision based on what makes you feel most comfortable.

We work to earn a living to support our lifestyle and part of that lifestyle is the home that we live in. If you start looking at a home as an investment, it will drive both you and your spouse crazy. You will always find reasons for not purchasing the home as an investment even though it fulfills a specific criterion that you have laid out or what you would want in your living environment.

Whether to buy or rent a home depends on how long you will be living there. If you will be living in the home for a number of years, then it probably makes sense to purchase the home outright since the ability to own your home will increase your feeling of well-being and stability and will allow you to reap the rewards of keeping your home in good repair.

If you plan on living in an area for a short period, for example, during residency, etc., then it is a best to rent, saving the difference toward accumulating money for a down payment on a home. Although there are many methods of figuring out whether it makes more sense economically to buy or rent a home, I find generally that most people like the stability of owning their own home over renting. Thus, I do not feel it is a good idea to make owning or renting a financial decision. Home ownership should be an attitudinal or emotional decision. Naturally, if you don't like the idea of being tied down to owning a home, then renting or leasing may be best for you.

History shows that owning a home has worked out to be a very fine investment. Home ownership can help you build net worth. It is my partiality to recommend that my clients purchase their home. However, you should purchase or build a home specifically to your needs, not buy a bigger house because it will have better resale nor should you buy a smaller house because you are afraid to spend the extra $200 or $300 a month in mortgage payments. Buy to fulfill your needs.

When buying it is best to put as small an amount of money down as possible and to finance the home over as long a period of time as you can (i.e., a 30-year fixed rate mortgage). If you go with a mortgage that is not a fixed rate loan, you should negotiate a interest rate cap so you have a guarantee from the financial institution that the rate would not go over 14 or 15 percent, etc. An interest rate cap gives you predictability and helps assure you that your payment will not go through the roof.

Future chapters of this book illustrate that a key to financial planning is to have balance in both your lifestyle and your business style. To take all of your money and have it go toward home mortgage payments can be financially unwise, so don't lock yourself into a short-term 10–15 year mortgage.

The chapters on budgeting should help you with being sure that you do not get financially strapped by home mortgage payments; however, a good rule is to keep your mortgage payments and housing costs at less than 35 percent of your gross income to allow you to live a balanced lifestyle; save some money toward the future; build net worth; educate the children, etc.

When purchasing a second home or resort property this also should be purchased specifically for lifestyle reasons. Generally the economics will not work out on purchasing a cottage or a second home because after figuring mortgage payments, cost of the down payment, the taxes, and the maintenance on that property, it usually is best to rent. More and more people do purchase second homes because they like the idea of having the permanency of a place to go. If you decide that owning is best for you, then you should avoid buying a $100,000 condo because you think it will have better resale value than the $50,000 condo that will fulfill your needs adequately. If you are thinking about purchasing a time share property, my specific advice is *don't*. Generally time shares are a very poor deal over any of the alternatives, i.e., owning the whole property or renting. The deals that I've seen have been a rip off and the sellers that promote such deals should wear masks.

If you are thinking of selling your home using realtors or selling a piece of property, Table 4-1 is a checklist to help you in appraising your needs, finding a realtor, and analyzing whether that realtor can help you sell your home.

You will notice that I have a strong partiality toward having an experienced, honest, successful, full-time career-oriented realtor as the marketing professional for your home. This is not to say that you should not consider first selling your home on your own in a "For Sale by Owner" situation. I am saying that if you decide to use a realtor that you do choose the best. The guidelines in Table 4-1 should assist you in making this decision.

The average person moves about every 5–7 years and because of this you will probably be selling 5–10 houses during your lifetime. Each of these home sales will be a major financial transaction for you. It is very important that you get top dollar for your home and that you minimize all costs associated with selling your home. It is often not hard to sell your home on your own; however, if you don't have the time or the temperament, you should choose a realtor. Also, a realtor can help you when purchasing a home. For example, if you have two subdivisions with homes that you like equally, a realtor may say, purchase your home in Subdivision A because its homes have a history of increasing in value, while Subdivision B may be having a new paper processing plant moving in right next door, which could drastically reduce the values of your prospective homes, since the odor and noise from the plant might be unpleasant.

In addition, a savvy realtor can help you with financing, making a decision on whether to buy or rent, and help refer you to a competent attorney to help you with any legal documents that must be reviewed on your real estate transactions.

YOUR OFFICE

Choosing where to locate your office should be based on only one important criterion: location for your clients' convenience. Your office should be easy to find, have adequate parking, and if possible, stand alone so that its location can also serve as an advertisement for your practice. Although, naturally you should keep your cost of your office location reasonable, spending $1 or $2 more per square foot to have a very convenient location should not be a consideration when choosing where to put your office.

Whether to purchase or rent your office should be a separate and distinct decision. However, I think that the best investment that a physician can make in real estate, is the office building that will house his or her

Table 4-1
Selling Your Home
_____

What to look for in your realtor.

Your realtor should be:
1. Experienced and honest.
2. Prove his or her competence.
3. Full time and career oriented.
4. Successful.
5. Professional in attitude and appearance.
6. Aggressive.
7. Up-to-date on new marketing methods and the real estate business.

Your realtor should:
1. Give you a written appraisal with a written method of how he or she came to the specific price to charge for your home.
2. Give you a written marketing plan of action on how he or she will market your home (i.e., open houses, newspaper ads, brochures, etc.)
3. Give you a list of references that you can call.
4. Go over a home appearance checklist with you to help make your home more marketable.

Your real estate agent's firm should:
1. Be a member of the multiple listing service.
2. Be reputable and serve your local area.
3. Be career oriented—hiring only full-time career professionals.
4. If you are in major metropolitan areas such as New York, Chicago, Detroit, Los Angeles, etc., your real estate firm should have a local and national network referral service.

You should:
1. Feel 100 percent comfortable with your realtor and his or her firm.
2. Not be present at personal showings or open houses.
3. Complete tasks highlighted from home appearance checklist (i.e., keep lawn mowed, fresh flowers, fix water marks, etc.).
4. Consider selling your house on your own before listing it if you or your spouse has the time and temperament. You can hire a competent real estate appraiser and lawyer to help.
5. Read over a listing agreement carefully before signing and make sure you write in exceptions to the listing of people who you may have as prospects and list built-in items affixed to your home that you want to keep (i.e., bar, chandelier, bookshelves, desk, light fixtures, etc.).
6. Have a lawyer review all closing documents regarding all your real estate transactions prior to closing.
_____

Source: Kimberly Sutherland, Signature Realty, Suttons Bay, MI. With permission.

practice, since you will know the tenant, take good care of the environment, and be able to build to suit your specific needs. My advice to clients who are considering getting investment real estate is to first look at building or purchasing their own office building. However, before you purchase your office building you should make sure that you are satisfied and comfortable with the area that you are practicing in and that you are comfortable with the type of practice that you have (i.e., few associates, a sole practioner, etc.).

Owning your own office building as with any real estate investment has a number of advantages: (1) tax advantages, (2) inflation hedge, (3) equity build-up through paying down on a mortgage, (4) any outlays made to improve or maintain the building will benefit you the owner, and (5) since you are the owner and tenant, you will be assured of having a top quality tenant.

The primary disadvantages that have to do with owning your office are: (1) lack of liquidity; (2) inability to meet the mortgage payments; (3) being tied down to that location if you decided to move; (4) property values could go down; and (5) tax laws could change.

If you are considering real estate purchase for investment reasons then you should analyze real estate as you would other investments. However, real estate has a tendency to be a little bit more complicated because its tax benefits complicate the methodologies of analyzing real estate investments.

One of the best methods of analyzing real estate investments is to pretend that the real estate investment has no tax benefits whatsoever, and that you are putting 100 percent of the purchase price into the property (i.e., buying the property for all cash). If a real estate deal looks very favorable without the tax and benefits of leverage (i.e., debt) to finance the property, then you probably have a project that has merits for further consideration as an investment.

Many physicians purchase real estate not for an investment but as a tax shelter. You should never purchase real estate as a tax shelter; you should purchase real estate only if you feel it will make you money in excess of the rates of return that you could receive on other investments. Some people have become very wealthy through real estate investments, while others have ruined their financial situation because of improper use of real estate. As with any investment, you should diversify your real estate holdings and make sure that you do not purchase any one deal that could harm you financially if it turned out to be a complete loser as an investment.

If you do not have a significant amount of cash to invest in real estate then use a partnership and purchase just a piece of the action. There is no excuse and no reason for jeopardizing your financial health because you could "get rich quick" through some real estate deal. Remember "If it sounds too good to be true, it probably is."

Table 4-2 illustrates some methods of figuring the rate of return on real estate investments. Even though the example is oversimplified, it is a good

Table 4-2
Figuring Return on a Real Estate Investment

	$100,000 Investment			
EXAMPLE # 1				
Cash flow*	@ $	1,000.	=	1.0 %
Net tax benefits †	@ $	5,600.	=	5.6 %
Principal reduction	@ $	500.	=	0.5 %
Appreciation	@ $	10,000.	=	10.0 %
Totals	$	17,100.	=	16.6 %
EXAMPLE # 2				
Cash flow*	- @ $	5,000.	=	-5.0 %
Net tax benefits	@ $	10,000.	=	10.0 %
Principal reduction	@ $	500.	=	0.5 %
Appreciation	@ $	2,000.	=	2.0 %
Totals	$	12,500.	=	12.0 %
EXAMPLE # 3				
Cash flow*	- @ $	5,000.	=	5.0 %
Net tax benefits	@ $	5,000.	=	5.6 %
Principal reduction	@ $	500.	=	0.5 %
Decrease in value	- @ $	10,000.	=	-10.0 %
Totals	- $	5,500.	=	6.10 %

* After debt service, real estate taxes, insurance, and all costs associated with property.
† Net tax benefit, i.e., $ 20,000 depreciation in a 28% bracket ($ 20,000 x 28 % = $ 5,600).

If looking at a property proforma you should expect a minimum of 8% to 10% net annual return from all sources exclusive of price appreciation—price appreciation should be your gravy.

starting point. It is best when considering real estate investments to have another real estate professional, or a financial planner, accountant, or attorney familiar with real estate review the specific transaction in which you are thinking about involving yourself. The final decision is yours, however, if they gave you some negatives about the property or the project; you will know them before going into the project so you will be able to handle any contingency (i.e., balloon payments on debt, lack of total occupancy, zoning problems).

This book and this chapter does not have a goal of giving you a complete understanding of real estate. If you are considering purchasing individual real estate as an investment for yourself, you should read some books on real estate. Also, there are many fine professionals out there who can help you. These experts and professionals should be hired just as you would hire other professionals using the guidelines in the chapters in this book on hiring professionals.

If you plan on buying a great deal of real estate, get your real estate license in your state so you at least have some basic knowledge of real estate and the laws affecting real estate. If you do not have the time to get involved, you might consider using other professionals or have your spouse get licensed if they are so inclined.

RECOMMENDED READING

Harrison HS: Houses. Chicago, National Association of Realtors, 1973

Real Estate Desk Book. Englewood Cliffs, NJ, Institute for Business Planning, Inc., 1979

Semenow RW: Questions and Answers on Real Estate. Englewood Cliffs, NJ, Prentice-Hall, Inc., 1948

5

I Hate Budgets

Having worked in the financial industry for over 10 years, I have found that I started out not liking budgets and I still do not like working with clients on budgeting.

As a physician/businessperson, and also as a person who runs your family household finances, it is important that you know what your family income sources are and where your money is going. This process of income and expense monitoring allows you to see what "fat" can be trimmed from your expenses and what extra surpluses you have that could be utilized toward wealth creation or improving your lifestyle.

The starting point for setting up a budget is to fill out a budget sheet that shows your income and your monthly expenses. You should monitor your monthly expenses for a few months so that you can get a feel for where your money is going and where it is coming from. Figure 5-1 is a budget sheet that you can fill out at your leisure on where your money is coming from and going. It is best to use the budget form for a few months so that you can get a feel for where your money goes.

It is my belief that most people tend to be prudent about their monthly expenses and tend to live within their means. However, often things will askew a budget such as some financial trauma, children's education, purchasing a new house, an office building, or an investment with improperly structured debt, etc. This chapter will also deal with the proper use of debt as a methodology of increasing spendable income so that more money can go toward supporting yourself and/or creating wealth.

It is a good idea to monitor your income and expenses for a 3-month period. Sometimes monitoring them over different months is helpful, if your expenses tend to be cyclical, i.e., greater expenses in the summer because of vacation and travel. After you have completed your budget for a 3-month period, then estimate your average expenses for the month (the personal budget worksheet helps you with this as it has a column for that contingency).

You will notice on the personal budget sheet that the amount left to invest after income taxes is put in a place other than as a monthly expense. The reason for this is to help you realize that the way you invest your money should be tax efficient, i.e., using IRAs, retirement plan trusts,

		1st Month	2nd Month	3rd Month	Monthly Average
INCOME					
Total Monthly Earnings	@	_____	_____	_____	_____
MONTHLY EXPENSES (fixed)					
House/rent payments*	@	_____	_____	_____	_____
Home insurance ÷ 12	@	_____	_____	_____	_____
Property taxes ÷12	@	_____	_____	_____	_____
Car payment #1*	@	_____	_____	_____	_____
Car payment #2*	@	_____	_____	_____	_____
Car Expenses	@	_____	_____	_____	_____
Phone (personal)	@	_____	_____	_____	_____
Electricity (pesonal)	@	_____	_____	_____	_____
Gas, oil (heat)	@	_____	_____	_____	_____
Food	@	_____	_____	_____	_____
Child care	@	_____	_____	_____	_____
Entertainment	@	_____	_____	_____	_____
Travel-vacations	@	_____	_____	_____	_____
Life insurance	@	_____	_____	_____	_____
Disability Insurance	@	_____	_____	_____	_____
Health insurance	@	_____	_____	_____	_____
Cottage or 2nd home*	@	_____	_____	_____	_____
Net investment expenses	@	_____	_____	_____	_____
Home maintenance	@	_____	_____	_____	_____
Credit card	@	_____	_____	_____	_____
Credit card	@	_____	_____	_____	_____
Other	@	_____	_____	_____	_____
Other	@	_____	_____	_____	_____
Other	@	_____	_____	_____	_____
Other	@	_____	_____	_____	_____
Other	@	_____	_____	_____	_____
TOTALS	@	═══════	═══════	═══════	═══════
(A) Amount left to invest and for income taxes	@	_____	_____	_____	_____
(B) Income taxes	@	_____	_____	_____	_____
(C) Surplus Deficit**		_____	_____	_____	_____

Total Debts @ $ _____

*Total monthly debt payments for above   -$ _____.
**Subtract (B) from (A) to get Surplus/Deficit (C).

Fig. 5-1. Personal budget sheet.

proper business form, etc., as we have, and will discuss in other chapters of this book. Note, however, that it is still necessary to write down the amount that you paid for income taxes for that 3-month period. Also note that there is a place to put your total debts and total monthly debt payments from your personal budget worksheet. This is because the two areas of budget that I see clients get very out of balance on are income taxes and debt management.

You will find that it is inconvenient and hard to change your monthly fixed expenses, other than to rearrange debt and/or taxes. I find that most people live their lives prudently, and I do not believe that it's good to change your lifestyle drastically, unless you have a specific goal in mind that you feel is worth the sacrifice of having less money going to entertainment or travel, etc. Thus, this chapter will concentrate on proper use of debt management, and although it will not address specific tax planning, other chapters in this book will. You should come back to the budget sheet after you are wiser about the proper use of tax management and see what can be done to reduce your taxes and increase the amount of money going for wealth creation or lifestyle.

The key to debt management is to have your debt so that the required payments are spread over the longest term at the lowest interest rate. Many physicians, especially young physicians, find themselves significantly in debt with large debt payments on short-term loans. This short term debt, coupled with high taxes and tremendous consumer spending, i.e., purchasing your first refrigerator, first couch, outfitting an office, your home or apartment, etc., causes a young physician to be constantly broke and often they will find themselves with a lot of anxiety caused by excessive debt payments and taxes. What is important to understand, is that your income will be consistent and significant, and thus you should manage your debt in a methodology that realizes that you have a 30–40 year practice life, and that there is nothing wrong with spreading your payments out over a long period of time. To spread payments out, however, you have to trust yourself, and only use debt where necessary to significantly increase lifestyle or to help further or start up a practice.

Figure 5-2 is a worksheet that you should complete, listing everything about your debt situation. This worksheet can help you to see whether rearranging your debt can make sense. On the sample financial plan it shows an illustration of rearranging debt that you may find helpful as it rearranges debt in a more wholistic manner, rather than looking specifically at debt through a microscope as a debt management worksheet does.

Most people do not manage their debt, nor do they analyze their debt to see what is the best way to structure it. Usually debt is acquired because of some financial trauma, or to purchase an asset, i.e., purchase a home, a cottage, a car, a boat, to pay last years' income taxes , etc. After awhile an

Debt Type	Asset Value	Debt Principal Amount	Monthly Payment	Debt Interest Rate	Year of Balloon On Debt?	Loan Period
Home	——	——	——	——	——	——
Cottage	——	——	——	——	——	——
Car #1	——	——	——	——	——	——
Car #2	——	——	——	——	——	——
School	——	——	——	——	——	——
Office Equipment	——	——	——	——	——	——
Bank Note #1	——	——	——	——	——	——
Bank Note #2	——	——	——	——	——	——
Credit Cards	——	——	——	——	——	——
Other	——	——	——	——	——	——
Other	——	——	——	——	——	——
Totals	——	——				

Goals: (1) Spread required payments over longest period possible. (2) Do not borrow yourself into hole with new found spending power.

Steps: (1) Borrow against home equity for long period. (2) Pay off highest debt payment to debt amount first, regardless of interest rate. (3) Work with your banker to re-schedule your payment over a longer period. (4) Understand that principal reduction is an inefficient way to create wealth and build net worth. Put your principal payment into your I.R.A. and Pension Plan.

A

Fig. 5.2. (*Continues*).

Debt Type	Asset Value	Debt Principal Amount	Monthly Payment	Debt Interest Rate	Year of Balloon On Debt?	Loan Period
Home	$125,000.	$ 80,000.	1,215.	13%	N/A	15 Years
Cottage	N/A					
Car #1	12,000.	10,000.	271.	12½%	N/A	5 Years
Car #2	5,000.	1,000.	90.	10%	N/A	1 Year
Office Equipment	25,000.	20,000.	510.	10%	N/A	5 Years
Bank Note*	N/A	15,000.	500.	Prime + 2%	1 Year	Renews
Credit Card Visa		3,000.	100.	18%	N/A	N/A
Credit Card Mastercard		3,500.	110.	18%	N/A	N/A
Other Parents (School)		5,000.	200.	None	None	2 Years
Totals	$137,500.	$137,500.	2,996.	Varies	Varies	Varies

*To pay prior 2 years' taxes

Steps: (1) Borrow maximum against home for long period Usually can borrow 80% of value, $125,000. x 80% = $100,000. = $1,098./monthly payment at 10.5% for 30 years. $100,000. - $80,000. to pay off existing mortgage = $20,000. to use for Step 2. (2) Pay off high payment to debt amount loans first, regardless of interest rate:

	Debt	Monthly Payment
Car #2	$1,000.	$ 90.
Visa	3,000.	100.
Mastercard	3,500.	110.
Parents	5,000.	200.
Total	$12,500.	$ 500.

Fig. 5.2. (*Continues*).

39

(3) Pay down bank note at $7,500 ($7,500. left after step 2). (4) Call loan officer and request ability to pay bank loans off for equipment and note over 7 years at 12% = monthly payment of $582.

New Debt Schedule

Debt	Debt Amount	Payment	Interest	Loan Period
Home	$100,000.	1,098.	10.5%	30 years
Equipment and note	27,500.	582.	12%	7 Years
Car #1	10,000.	271.	12.5%	5 Years
	137,000.	1,951.	Various	Various

Old Payment at $2,996.—New Payment at $1,951. = Savings of $1,045./Monthly.

B

Fig. 5-2. (*Continued*) (A) Debt management worksheet. (B) Sample debt management worksheet.

individual can often end up with a mish-mash of unmanaged debt that is counter-productive to achieving the goals of accumulating wealth, or just efficiently managing loan payments.

Keep in mind that the improper use of debt can raise tremendous havoc for an individual, and it can ruin years of well-laid plans if not properly managed. Avoid using debt to make investments that have significant risk or where the income from the investment is supposed to pay the debt payment back. For example, if you purchase an apartment complex with a loan that has a debt service of $1,000/month, you should not assume that the income from your project will pay that debt. You should be able to handle the $1,000 monthly debt service on your own, exclusive of the income from the property.

While this approach is very conservative and will tend to make a few real estate agents mad, you should avoid accumulating debt service that you cannot handle 100 percent out of your personal service income. Naturally, whenever you use debt to make an investment, or for any other purpose, you should have adequate disability income insurance, so that if you were to be disabled you would have enough income from your disability policy to pay your debt service, plus provide an income to maintain your lifestyle. The chapter on insurance covers this in greater detail.

In dealing with banks or other lending institutions, always go into the bank knowing what you want, what you will be assigning to the bank as collateral, and how you plan on paying that loan back. If you are wondering how to structure your debt, use the worksheet in this chapter and ask a loan officer for his or her advice. You should know specifically how you will pay the money back, and why it is a good deal for that bank to loan you money. Banks are in the business of loaning money—that is a service that they provide. They need to make loans in order to afford to pay dividends and create profits for their corporation. You should have a good positive relationship with your bank. Never work with a banker that bullies you, is abusive, or does not hold your situation in strict confidence. Also, never lie to your banker, or do anything other than what you tell the bank that you will do. Since bankers make decisions on your credit, character, collateral, and cash flow (the four Cs of banking), you want to make sure that you take every safeguard to protect your ability to borrow money.

Even if you have excellent or excess cash flow, and feel no monthly pinch in making your monthly budget, you still should go through the debt management and budgetary process to see if there is any way that you could increase your spendable income, or your ability to create net worth for yourself through proper debt management.

On an annual basis, your accountant will be needing specific information on your tax situation. When you are set up in practice, you should sit down with your accountant and go over how you will keep your records and books in order for him or her to be able to complete your tax returns.

Records that should be kept permanently are:
Stock and bond transactions; corporate P.C. records, minutes, etc.; titles, mortgages, etc.; year-end ledgers and trial balances; insurance inspections reports; tax records and returns; fixed assets appraisals; earnings records; W-4 forms; cancelled checks; inventory and equipment records; excise tax information; financial statements; legal and important papers and correspondence.

Records that should be kept for 7 years are:
Deposit books and stubs; outstanding checks and draft records; cancelled payroll checks; bank statements after audit; accounts payable ledgers; paid bills and vouchers; bids and offers; purchase contracts; expired leases; payroll journals and summaries; time cards and paychecks; payroll deduction records; uncollected accounts files; expired contracts with customers; cancelled notes; expired contracts and agreements; insurance records.

Records that should be kept for 3 years are:
Daily or periodic cash reports; petty cash vouchers; purchase orders of confirmed purchases; fidelity bonds records and records of insurance policies in force; trial balances (for receivables and payables); invoices; credit classifications and ratings; W-2 forms; garnish and assignments on wages.

Monthly trial balances should be kept for a period of 5 years and general correspondence should be kept for a period of 1–5 years, at your discretion.

Fig. 5-3. Records checklist.

Do not wait until April 14th of your first year to see an accountant. You should see a competent accountant right away so that he or she can set you on the right road to proper record keeping.

In addition to keeping tax records for your accountant on an annual basis, there are many records that will need to be kept permanently or for a number of years. Figure 5-3 lists what records you should keep and for how long. You should use this as a guide in your own record keeping.

6
Risk Management Strategies

A cornerstone to any financial plan is the proper management of risk. Proper risk management is essential. It is the most important area of financial planning. It is also the most misunderstood. Risk management is the knowledge that various risks exist and the evaluation of the magnitude and effects that those risks could have upon you and your financial well-being.

The first steps to take in proper risk management is to analyze the risks that you have and to evaluate those risks to see how they should be handled. There are four risk management techniques that can be used.

First is the avoidance of the risk (which simply means to avoid the possible risk). For example, choosing not to drive on icy, snowy roads would be a method of avoiding risk, as would the decision to not allow your children to swim in a swimming pool unsupervised by an adult.

The second method of risk management is risk minimization or reduction. As a physician you are practicing this methodology of risk management with many of your patients, telling them to avoid smoking, avoid certain types of food, etc.

Putting a sprinkler system in your office does not reduce the risk of a fire occurring; however, it does reduce the risk that fire could destroy your records and equipment. Throwing a snow shovel, bag of sand, some warm mittens, and boots in your car before driving during a snowstorm reduces your risk of spending the night in a snowdrift.

Accepting the risk is the third method used by risk managers. Many risks are minor and their effect on your financial well-being would be modest, such as the risk that your milk will sour in the refrigerator or the risk your car won't start. It would be foolish to insure yourself against such risks since most of these risks will happen and the cost of loss is modest. However, certain risks must be retained such as the risk of loss because of war or riot.

When most people think of risk management they think of insurance. Insurance is the fourth method of risk management. It deals with the transfer of risk. Transfer of risk consists of any methodology that you use that transfers the risk that you have to someone else. For example, having a patient sign a form stating that they will hold you harmless prior to a surgery is a method of avoiding a risk of lawsuit. Your liability is at least partially transferred in that method. Perhaps a better method would be the complete transfer of the risk and that would be through the purchase of malpractice insurance. Insurance is definitely the most important type of transfer device and constitutes transferring the risk to a third party, i.e., an insurance company in return for payment of an insurance premium.

For most of this chapter we will deal with the utilization of insurance in transferring risk. Insurance is a means of reducing or limiting a risk by dividing the risk of loss among many individuals. The most important consideration (in purchasing insurance to transfer your risk) is that you should only transfer risks that you can not handle. You should not insure against risks that are predictable and whose financial effect on you would be modest, such as the risk of needing new eyeglasses, or your teeth polished, filled, or drilled, etc. Also, you should only insure against big expenses and use deductibles and other cost-sharing methods to help reduce the cost of insurance. For example, there is tremendous savings in purchasing car insurance by taking a $500 or $1,000 additional risk in the deductible. It is foolish and a waste of money to insure against expenses that you could handle. Whenever you pay a premium to an insurance company, they take a piece of the action to cover commissions, accounting, administration, marketing expenses, and other overhead expenses. Thus they can only give you back a percent of your premium for the assumption of the risk. If you can handle, for example, a $500 bill, then you should have a $500 deductible on your car insurance. However, it would be foolish to have the first $500 of auto expenses covered and nothing over the $500.

What you need to worry about in purchasing car insurance or other insurance is the $10,000, $100,000, $1,000,000 expenses, not the small, modest, predictable expenses. You should assume these small expenses and have a sum of money set aside to use to pay for small losses that come along that are not covered by insurance.

Since insurance agents are paid commissions based on the premium income they bring into their insurance companies, there is a conflict of interest in their advising you as to the best method of purchasing insurance. Thus, often they will advise you to have a modest or no deductible policy which may cost $1,000, while a $500 deductible policy would reduce your cost to perhaps $600 or $700 on the same policy.

Buying property and liability insurance is important to your financial security. When purchasing property insurance you must decide what the possible losses would be that you could incur by owning a given piece of property, such as a home. Then you have to decide what kind of insurance best covers the risks that you assume from ownership of the property, how much insurance you should have, and, lastly, what insurer or insurers you should use to provide this coverage.The key, mentioned earlier, to buying insurance is to only cover substantial risk, i.e., the risk you cannot handle.

Choosing a good insurance agent is very important as policies are very complicated. It is best to tell your agent that you wish to have a policy that will cover you against the risks that are substantial, no matter how remote that risk may be, while not covering you for the smaller risks, such as breakage of a window, or risks of under $1,000 or so. The first thing to ask your agent when purchasing insurance is what risks will the policy not cover, i.e., what risks will you be assuming, which risks are being transferred, and which are not. You can then decide whether the risks you will be assuming are ones that you can handle by yourself. If they cannot be handled, you should transfer those risks to the insurance company. Following is a detailed list that shows what you should look for when purchasing homeowners insurance, automobile insurance, and umbrella liability coverage.

PROPERTY AND CASUALTY INSURANCE FOR DOCTORS

Auto

1. *Bodily injury liability limits.* Be sure you carry at least $300,000 limit (any lawsuit in Michigan is over $100,000). Then purchase a personal liability umbrella for at least $1,000,000–$5,000,000 to protect against lawsuit in excess of the basic auto policy limit of $300,000. This covers you if your negligence causes injury or death to another party via vehicular accident.

2. *Physical damage coverage.* Insures the value of your car. This includes (1) comprehensive coverage—such losses as a stone hitting and breaking a windshield, fire, theft, vandalism, hitting a deer or fowl, a tree falling on your car and so forth; (2) collision—You hit another car, person, or object, or your vehicle is hit by another vehicle. You are considered at fault, if your action or failure to take action was over 50 percent of the cause of the accident. There are three forms of collision coverage: (a) *broad form* (the best)—You pay no deductible regardless of fault. (b) *basic or standard or regular collision*—You pay a deductible regardless of fault. If not at fault, you may be able to recover your deductible from the other driver through legal action. (The limit for recovery in Michigan is $400.) (c) *limited collision*—pays no benefit if you are at fault. If not at fault, the other driver must be identified or you must have witnesses if a hit-and-run. This form of collision is generally not recommended.

When purchasing physical damage coverage you will have a choice of deductibles. The deductible amount chosen is subtracted from the payment made in the event of a loss and you are paid the difference in amount of the loss. We generally advise a $50 deductible on comprehensive coverage, and a $500 to $1,000 deductible on collision coverage. The key to selecting a deductible amount involves the individual's ability to pay and risk of loss. The higher the deductible, the lower the premium. A person can generally take higher deductibles if he or she can afford the out-of-pocket expenses in the event of a loss. Also, a person who is a good driver and lives in a low-risk area can generally do better with higher deductibles. A low-risk area is an area where there is seldom a problem with auto theft (rural areas—not large cities like Detroit, or poor areas of town, vehicle seldom unattended— lots of cars stolen from airport parking lots, from city streets overnight, and so forth). If you drive on gravel or poor roads, the odds of a rock damaging your car are high. High traffic areas are more prone to have many collisions.

Physical damage coverage is required when the vehicle is leased or financed. The leasing company or finance company may stipulate the maximum deductible amount they will allow.

3. *Uninsured/underinsured motorist coverage.* Uninsured motorist coverage is in the event that you suffer a bodily injury and the other driver or vehicle is not insured—you can sue through your own insurance for financial compensation. Underinsured motorist—in the event you suffer a bodily injury and the other driver's vehicle's insurance liability limits are low, you can sue through your own company for higher limits.

Uninsured and underinsured motorist coverages are optional. Basic limits are $20,000 per person/$40,000 per occurrence. We advise limits of $100,000 per person/$300,000 per occurrence. Underinsured motorist coverage must exceed the $20,000/$40,000 limit to be of any benefit, as in Michigan, for example, the law states you must carry Bodily Injury and Property Damage liability limits of at least $20,000 per person/$40,000 per occurrence and $10,000 property damage on any auto policy you carry.

4. *Personal injury protection.* This coverage is what no-fault insurance is all about. It consists of two coverages: medical expenses and wage loss.

A key area of concern for persons with high income is to take "Full Wage Loss Benefit," as the no-fault wage loss maximum in Michigan is $2,624 per month (1985—approximate figure). If you elect excess wage loss coverage, your own disability programs pay first and then the no-fault pays up to, but not exceeding, the current maximum limit. If a person elects full coverage—first the no-fault coverage pays the maximum a person is eligible to (varies according to income up to the maximum $2,624/no limit), then your private disability coverage pays on top of the no-fault limit. You can get both.

There is much more to auto insurance, but these are the key areas and they involve choices by the insured as to limits of liability, deductibles, and coverage options. The other areas of auto insurance are mandatory on a basic policy.

Here are some optional coverages to consider:

1. *Road service/towing and labor.* Reimbursement for breakdown. (Service— towing, emergency help—not parts or mechanic's bill.) Amounts payable and cost of coverage varies by company.
2. *Rental reimbursement.* Pays you for a rental car if yours is stolen or disabled and in shop or totaled after an accident. Does not cover breakdown/repair time.
3. *Accessories coverage.* For extras such as stereo, CB, radar detectors that are not a permanent part of the car (automatically covered if in "dash"). Tapes still not covered. Camper tops and caps on a pick-up should be listed when insuring the vehicle to be sure they are covered.

     Other things/provisions: Always read the policy and ask your agent if you have questions.
   - Who is insured?
   - Substitute vehicle provisions (rented/borrowed car)
   - Exclusions (letting unlicensed driver use car, letting impaired/intoxicated person use car—voids coverage).
   - Always know what is not covered, why it isn't covered, and can it be! Ask your agent—compare between companies.
   - Contracts vary and so does level of knowledge among agents.

Most importantly, ask your agent if there are additional questions!

Homeowners Coverage

When you own the building, there are three basic forms of building coverage.

1. HO-1. Named peril—covering fire, lightning, and removal (never get form 1.)
2. HO-2. Sometimes called "broad" coverages—named peril:
   - fire—fire, lightning, removal
   - extended coverage—windstorm, hail, smoke, explosion, riot, riot attending a strike, civil commotion, aircraft, and vehicles
   - optional perils—breakage of glass, falling objects, weight of ice and snow, sleet, limited water damage, and building collapse
   - V & MM—vandalism and malicious mischief. (Form 2 is common, but not worth the savings in premium compared with form 3.)
3. HO-3. Called special or "all risk" coverage. This is the best form. Covers for all risk of physical damage, subject to standard exclusions. Standard exclusions are flood, war, nuclear explosion, earthquake,

neglect of the insured to use all reasonable means to save and preserve the property at and after a loss, and more. Refer to lines 7–24 of a standard fire policy form for exact wording and exclusions.

Contents Coverage

Contents are covered for the perils listed in form 1 and form 2 of building coverage, not for form 3 coverages.

One's best bet is to read the policy for exact terms and conditions and limitations of coverage. Then ask your agent how to cover the gaps.

Limitations on contents coverage. As I mentioned earlier, contents are covered for form 2 perils on a standard contract. Most items are alright this way. Items with limitations on coverage in almost all homeowners and tenant homeowner contracts: jewelry (usually $500 limit), furs, fine arts, silverware, coins, stamps, guns, money, precious metals, securities, manuscripts, camera equipment, musical instruments, boats, and RVs and their equipment. These items can all be insured on a specific basis under floaters or Inland Marine Policies.

Recommended Optional Coverages

(1) Scheduled equipment; (2) Inland marine coverage; (3) Mysterious disappearance (i.e., get home at night and the stove is gone, etc.); (4) Replacement cost coverage for contents. Eliminates reduction in value for depreciation "new for old"; (5) Guaranteed home replacement (see what company offers); (6) Business pursuits coverage. Babysitting by kids, rummage sales, incidental activities that are not full time and generate under $2,000 per year income (generally); (7) Theft coverage extension. Covers your personal property while in your car or boat (subject to policy conditions); and (8) Increase personal liability limit from the standard $25,000 to $300,000 (plus have a personal liability unbrella policy for 1 to 5 million). For doctors—you need specific coverage for doctors equipment (black bag coverage) that you carry with you. This can be purchased on home or business policy with a floater!

Deductibles

- •$250 is generally the best buy (10–15 percent discount on basic premium)
- •$100 (applies to all building and contents losses per occurrence) is most common

Other Considerations

Homeowners form HO-4. Covers contents and personal liability and additional living expenses for tenants (rent a house or apartment).

Homeowners form HO-6. Condo owners coverage covers contents and liability. This can be confusing. Always read the condo association contract to see who is responsible for what. Condo insurance is complicated. Make sure you discuss with your agent what is covered and what is not and check out co-insurance amount carefully.

Umbrella Liability Coverage

Personal

Personal umbrella liability insurance goes on top of home and auto policy and provides catastrophic coverage—excess over the required underlying limit on the home and auto policy. (Home and auto limit must generally be $300,000 but this varies by company.) It also fills many cracks and loopholes in home and auto policies. It provides worldwide liability coverage, while home and auto policies do not.

Key Points

Do not buy umbrella that: (1) Uses "following form" coverage—follow form means it only pays if your home and auto policy pays first—won't cover the cracks and loopholes, won't provide worldwide coverage because the home and auto policies won't. (2) Says it will "reimburse" you for liability claim rather than "pay on behalf of." With reimbursement, you could have to pay first—most of us could not pay a $1,000,000 (or more or less) judgment in order to get reimbursed later. You want the insurance company to pay it for you.

Commercial Liability Umbrella

The Commercial Liability Umbrella is the same as above, except that it responds to business activities. A professional or business owner needs both umbrellas: Personal for coverage on top of home and auto policy, commercial for coverage on top of business liability policy.

Business Insurance

This subject is too detailed to explain fully here. However, following are some things to look out for: (1) Co-insurance clause (penalty if not insured at required minimum percent of value of property), (2) Deductibles—vary by your ability to self-insurance for small losses and difference in premium for higher deductibles and risk of loss (high or low exposure), (3) Supplemental coverages—valuable papers and records, loss of earnings, extra expense, overhead expense coverage, crime coverage, loss of rents, computer coverage (electronic data processsing policies), flood coverage, earthquake coverage, replacement cost vs. actual cash value coverage on building and equipment and contents, nonowned and hired auto coverage, glass and/or sign coverage, personal injury coverage (advertising, false arrest, wrongful entry, malicious prosecution, slander, libel, etc. may be picked up on comprehensive general liability—broad form endorsement), and more.

In addition to having good homeowners and automobile insurance it is a good idea to have a comprehensive personal liability coverage that covers exposure of loss through legal liabilities, such as your dog bites your neighbor, a mailman or a visitor slips and falls on your front sidewalk, or your neighbor's child falls into your swimming pool and drowns, etc. These lawsuits can run into the millions of dollars and you need a good, comprehensive, personal liability policy to cover these risks.

Personal liability coverage is especially important to you as a physician, since physicians are prime targets for lawsuits. Attorneys do go after physicians because physicians have higher than average income and net worths, and thus, usually have adequate assets to pay a claim.

There are many risks associated with being a physician and a great risk is that of being sued in the line of providing professional services to your patients and clients. There are two primary types of malpractice insurance—"occurrence" and "claims made" policies. Under the terms of an occurrence policy the insurer carries a perpetual liability for any negligence that may have occurred while that policy was in force. Under a claims made policy, the insurance company assumes a liability only if a claim is made, or the potential for a claim is filed before the policy's termination date. However, some claims made policies will cover claims that are filed after the policy has run out.

Regardless of the event, your policy should cover the attorney's fees, cost of expert witnesses, court costs, costs of gathering evidence, and any settlement. These costs should be covered even if the lawsuit is fraudulent. The average award has been going up substantially every year and it is estimated that the average malpractice insurance claim will soon be in excess of $200,000.

You should choose the best, most up-to-date, professional liability insurance you can buy and make sure that your policy will cover you adequately. In addition, make sure that any of your associates, or people that work for you, fill in for you during vacations, etc., have a good malpractice insurance policy. You should also do all that you can to minimize the risk of malpractice claims through proper communication with your patients and by making sure that you prudently run your practice in compliance with the standard procedures of your profession.

Lastly, it cannot be overemphasized that your policies should pay all legal costs incurred by defending yourself in a liability case. For example, you could win the case and lose the war by having thousands of dollars in attorney fees not covered by the policy. Read your policy carefully and make sure you understand it.

HEALTH INSURANCE

As a physician you are very aware of health care costs and it is very important that you have a comprehensive, major medical policy that covers reasonable and customary hospital and medical expense costs. Your policy should pay private or semi-private room charges, intensive care, burn and/or cardiac care unit expenses in full, for an unlimited number of days. Your policy should include a copayment and per year stop loss provision at whatever you feel you can handle, i.e., $5,000 or $10,000 a year out-of-pocket maximum cost, with full coverage for pre-existing conditions and a maximum limit of no less than $250,000 (a million dollars is more reasonable). Cancellation protection should be provided by the policy's contract.

You, your spouse, family members, and anyone that is dependent on you, should have adequate hospitalization insurance.

Often it makes a lot of sense to have at least a $500–$1,000 deductible on your policy to save on premium costs, since you can handle those risks and also, many of your health care needs can be provided by yourself or your colleagues at little or no cost.

As with all insurance policies, it is always wise to ask your insurance advisor for a list of the limitations of your policy and charges your policy will not cover. Standard policy exclusions would be war, self-inflicted injuries, medical expenses that had no costs, expenses covered by a V.A. hospital, etc.

Key Provisions that Your Health Insurance Policy Should Have

1. Reasonable and customary coverage of hospital and medical expenses
2. Full semi-private room coverage
3. Full intensive care, burn unit, cardiac care coverage to policy maximum—not for certain number of days
4. Per year payment and Stop/Loss Provisions at whatever level you feel you can handle, i.e., $1,000, $5,000, $10,000, etc.
5. Full coverage of pre-existing conditions
6. Minimum policy limit of $250,000, although $1,000,000 is much better.
7. Cancellation protection

LIFE INSURANCE

Physicians are the biggest purchasers of individual life insurance in the United States. As a group, they purchase tremendous amounts of life insurance. Most of this life insurance is purchased inefficiently. When purchasing life insurance, you should strive to purchase an adequate amount of insurance at the most cost-effective method possible. You should not purchase life insurance or any other insurance (or any financial service for that matter) because of a friendship or other nonfinancial reason. You should purchase the insurance because it is the best deal that you can get.

   The first step in purchasing life insurance is to decide whether you need insurance. You may not need insurance if you have no one that is or will be dependent on you, or if no one would be harmed financially by your death. If you do have people that would suffer financially from your death, it is very important that you purchase adequate life insurance.

   Figure 6-1 can be utilized to help you figure out whether you have a need for life insurance. On the worksheet you should list out any individual who would be harmed financially should you die, for example, your spouse or children. Then you must decide how much you want them to receive—not in a lump sum benefit, but to provide for the loss of income caused by your death.

   For example, if you have debts you wish to pay off at death, you should list the amount of debts, then list the amount of income you figure that your family would need in order to support their lifestyle. When figuring income for your family do not figure on minimum needs, rather calculate the expenses of supporting their lifestyle. If you have young children or a spouse who is not financially sophisticated, it is also important to decide how your life insurance proceeds will be managed and used after you die. To relieve your spouse or children of this money management burden (for example, if you want life insurance to provide an income to your family), you may want to set up a life insurance trust that will provide them with an adequate monthly income for the rest of their lives, or as long as you feel is necessary.

   Inflation will impact your family's income, so it is very important that you use low interest assumptions in your calculations. For example, $100,000 at a 12 percent interest rate will provide your family with a $12,000 annual income; however, 12 percent is a high rate of return and does not provide any money to be reinvested to help offset inflation. Inflation at a 7 percent rate would make it so that $12,000 a year income would only purchase $6,000 worth of goods and services in 10 years and only $3,000 for goods and services in 20 years. Thus, it is very important that you use a lower rate of return in your family's income trust so that some of the money can be reinvested to help offset inflation. If you are very young, it makes sense to use a 5 or 6 percent rate of return. If you are older or near retirement, you might want to use up to a 6–8 percent rate of return.

   Each person's situation is different. If you feel 6 percent is a reasonable rate and your goal is to provide your family with a $4,000 monthly income, to figure out how much life insurance or other assets your family would need at your death, take $4,000 and divide that by .005 (6 percent divided by 12) to find the amount of money your family will need to provide them with an income of $4,000 monthly ($4,000 divided by .005 = $800,000). Hopefully, your spouse will hire a money manager or you'll name one in your trust and your insurance proceeds will earn greater than 6 percent used in this assumption and thus, each year your family should get a raise to help offset inflation.

Death Insurance Worksheet

Step #1

List below who would suffer financially if you died. (Example: spouse, children, parents, business partner, charity, friend, sibling.)

Name   **List type of loss**
                                 (i.e., income, debt payback, family care, etc.)

_____   _____

_____   _____

_____   _____

Step #2

List specific degree of economic well-being you would desire for above listed people.

Monthly income to _____ of $ _____
                        (Name)

Monthly income to _____ of $ _____
                        (Name)

Pay off debts of $ _____ for _____
                                                        (Name)

Cash resource of $ _____ for _____
                                                        (Name)

Special cash to _____ of $ _____
                        (Name)   (Lump sum)

Step #3

Total monthly income desired @ $ _____ divided by .005* = $ _____.

Cash to pay off debts, mortgages, for cash reserves, and
special cash   Total $ _____.

Total assets needed to provide for above = $ _____.
*(A 6% interest rate is used so that excess earnings
can go to help offset inflation.)

        Total assets needed (from above) $ _____
        Less liquid assets you own and
        assets which could be made
        liquid $ _____
        Total insurance death benefit
        you need $ _____*

*Note: Once you have calculated your insurance needs make sure that you coordinate your insurance properly with your other assets, wills, and trusts. A good estate planning attorney should assist you.

Fig. 6-1. Death insurance worksheet. (From Golden Rule Association of Financial & Investment Management Group, Suttons Bay, MI. With permission.)

Having worked with a number of physicians over the years we find that physicians often buy their insurance based on budgetary factors rather than the needs of their family. This is because they do not understand that there are many types of life insurance. For example, generally you can purchase term, graded premium, or an adjustable policy at extremely low cost. At age 35 a male should be able to purchase life insurance for less than $1 per $1,000, so a $1,000,000 policy would cost under $1,000 a year. Somewhere under age 45 you should be able to purchase $1,000,000 for a couple thousand dollars a year, and a person under the age of 55 should be able to purchase a $1,000,000 policy for under $5,000.

Generally as we get older, our need for life insurance should diminish since our net worth will increase and our children grow to a point where they are not dependents.

If you will need insurance for 10 years or longer, you should consider an adjustable policy, as its total cost should be lower over a 10-year or longer period than term insurance. However, never, ever purchase less insurance than you need because of cost. There is nothing wrong with owning term insurance throughout your life and since most nonterm policies are very expensive, term insurance is usually the best way to go. There are a few companies, however, that have extremely low cost adjustable or universal life policies that will provide lower overall cost over a 10-year, or longer, period.

When you purchase insurance you should seek competent financial help from an insurance professional or a financial planner who puts your needs on level with his or her own. If you have a pension plan and feel that you will need insurance for 10 years it is often a good idea to purchase your life insurance through your pension plan. This allows you to deduct a substantial portion of your life insurance outlay while still providing your family with the much needed protection.

Keep in mind that the best insurance is the insurance that is in force on the day that you die. Purchase insurance that has the minimum "bells and whistles." Never buy accidental death and if someone suggests the accidental death rider to you, he or she is no professional—find a new insurance advisor, because accidental death insurance is gambling with your family's financial security on the 7 percent chance you will die of an accident. Table 6-1 illustrates costs of a very competitive adjustable term life insurance.

Never purchase deposit term insurance or minimum deposit or tax qualified whole life insurance policies. If an agent recommends these insurance policies, find a new agent. These policies tend to be extremely expensive and lock you into a long-term relationship with a company, on an assumption that you are purchasing an insurance policy at a very low overall cost. Usually the opposite is the case as these policies have extremely high front end costs and make it so that primarily the agent for the company benefits and not you. Carefully analyze your insurance

Table 6-1
Sample Non-Smoker Rates (Supplied by a mutual company founded in the 1880s with a history of providing low cost flexible insurance protection to *all* their policyholders past and present).

Age	Guaranteed Annually Renewable Convertible Term Premium per 1,000 500,000 band	Level Premium Adjustable Life (designed for low outlay and low net cost) Non-Smoker Rate Premium per 1,000 for minimum outlay outlay adjustable	Number of years policy will stay in force at stated premium assuming 8%	assuming 10%	Per $1,000 of Death Benefit cash value in 10 & 20 Years Assuming 8% returns on cash values 10 Years	20 Years
25	.90	2.30	Life	Life	$17.	$70.
30	.94	2.32	82	Life	$17.	$64.
35	.94	3.30	76	83	$26.	$73.
40	1.19	4.46	81	Life	$37.	$113.
45	1.66	6.64	84	83	$53.	$162.
55	3.87	13.63	85	Life	$109.	$264.
65	9.67	33.00	Life	Life	$250.	$662.

Notes: Adjustable premiums are guaranteed for 5 years, policy will stay in force as stated based on current mortality costs and greater than guaranteed interest rates. Adjustable life allows premiums and death benefit flexibility. You can raise or lower premiums or death benefit as your needs change without having to have new policies issued. If you start to accumulate large cash values as above you can substantially reduce your outlay by using dividends to reduce premiums or a number of different options.

policies' costs for the first, second, third, and fourth years, etc., to assure yourself that you understand the exact cost of policies. Generally it is best just to stick with a good yearly renewable term or variable or adjustable policy. Try to stick within the parameters outlined above.

In purchasing life insurance, it is usually best to have just one policy rather than a number of smaller policies. And if your policies are over 4 or 5 years old it is probably to your best advantage to cash in those policies and purchase new insurance, since the old policies probably are not as competitively priced as the newer policies. This is not always the case, however. It is extremely important that an analysis is done to assure yourself that dropping your old policies is to your definite advantage. A competent life insurance agent or financial planner familiar with life insurance can analyze the true costs of keeping the old policies over dropping and purchasing new ones. Often the old insurance company will change their policy through an upgrade program to a more competitive product. Although this is not always a good deal for you, it must be explored.

In choosing a life insurance company, it is best to choose a company that has an A or better rating for financial strength, and a company whose philosophy is to benefit all their policy holders both past and present. There are a number of fine mutual life insurance companies that have truly lived the philosophy of mutualism, which means that the policy holder owns the company and the company is there to serve them and not the stockholders. I have a strong partiality toward mutual insurance companies since history has shown that many mutual companies have given their clients lower costs than stock life insurance companies. This is not always true, however, as I know of a number of mutual companies whose executives should wear masks when they come to work each day. I also know of some stock or non-par life insurance companies whose policy net cost and integrity toward the policy holders is top drawer.

You should not get too caught up in the "which insurance company is best procedure." Your first decision is to decide how much life insurance you need and make sure you purchase enough and when in doubt, buy good quality, guaranteed annual renewable and covertible term insurance. Also if you choose to drop your old insurance policy and to buy a new one, make sure that you keep your old insurance policy in force until your new policy is approved, reviewed, and in force before you drop the old policy.

Following is a letter that you should write to your insurance agent when purchasing life insurance through him or her. Actually some of the questions will not pertain to your specific transaction; however, letters like this should be shown to him or her with a request for the answers to the questions in writing. The insurance check-up list (Fig. 6-2) is something you should review periodically to assure your life insurance is always adequate. You should review your coverage at least every 12–16 months.

Dear Life Insurance Agent:

I would like answers to the following questions in writing on your letterhead:

1. How did you arrive at the specific amount of life insurance that you have recommended I purchase?
2. Why have you or why have you not recommended that I purchase the waiver of premium option with my coverage?
3. Is this policy guaranteed renewable so I can keep this policy in force for the rest of my life?
4. What is the worst case premium limits that this policy cost could go to?
5. What is the best case that the company illustrates for premium history without having to have new medical exams in the ensuing years?
6. Does this policy build up cash values? And if so, how much based on a (1) guaranteed rate of return, (2) 4% rate of return, (3) 8% rate of return, and (4) a 10% rate of return?
7. What is the company's history on paying interest on the cash value of the insurance policy?
8. Is this policy a participating policy whereby it will participate in the excess earnings of the company or is it a guaranteed cost policy where the excess earnings will go to the insurance company and thus its shareholders?
9. What is my exact beneficiary designation, both primary and secondary? And why do you recommend its current designation? (For example beneficiary designation may be spouse if living, otherwise all children born of this marriage or legally adopted equally as shall be living.)
10. What is the proposed insurance company's financial strength rating by Best?
11. What other companies do you represent and did you consider when choosing an insurance company to place my insurance with?
12. Did you completely, honestly and accurately answer all questions on the contract's application as I answered them? And also could I see a copy of the application and medical form submitted to the insurance company so that I may review it to assure its accuracy?
13. When you were recommending that I drop other insurance companies, how did you determine that it makes sense to drop my old insurance policies to purchase new?
14. Will you take care of assisting me in surrendering my old insurance policies or are you going to be leaving this up to me? What safeguards do I have that my new policy will be in force before you start surrender procedures of my old policies?
15. If this is a policy purchased through my corporation under a split dollar arrangement or through my pension plan, who will provide me with the PS-58 pure term insurance costs on an annual basis so that I can supply them to my accountant?

Thank you for the above information. You assistance is very much appreciated.

Sincerely yours,

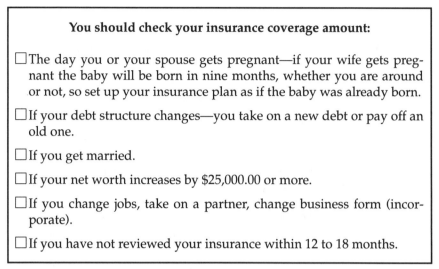

You should check your insurance coverage amount:

☐ The day you or your spouse gets pregnant—if your wife gets pregnant the baby will be born in nine months, whether you are around or not, so set up your insurance plan as if the baby was already born.

☐ If your debt structure changes—you take on a new debt or pay off an old one.

☐ If you get married.

☐ If your net worth increases by $25,000.00 or more.

☐ If you change jobs, take on a partner, change business form (incorporate).

☐ If you have not reviewed your insurance within 12 to 18 months.

Fig. 6-2. Death benefit insurance check-up list. (From Golden Rule Associates of Financial & Investment Management Group, Suttons Bay, MI. With permission.)

INCOME PROTECTION INSURANCE

Income protection or disability insurance is by far the most important insurance you, as a physician, can purchase. You are a money machine and your primary assets are your skills and your ability to utilize those skills. If you were unable to utilize your skills through sickness or accident, it would have a tremendous effect on your financial well-being, unless, of course, you are independently wealthy. There is a joke in the insurance industry that some disability policies are written with such tight limitations that "if you could sell pencils on street corners, you would not be considered disabled."

On the other end of contract provisions of disability policies is the policy that covers you for your specialty. These companies will pay full benefits if you are unable to practice your specialty, even if you are able to practice another specialty and earn the same or more money than before.

Before choosing a disability policy you first must decide whether you have a need for disability protection. Figure 6-3 may be utilized to help you decide how much disability income insurance you will need to support your lifestyle, and also help you decide what elimination period you should have on your policy.

An elimination period is the number of days you must wait before you receive a benefit from your policy. The limitation period generally runs from a 30-day wait, which has substantially greater cost, to a 1-year wait. The policy contract provisions are the most important elements you must look at when comparing disability policies.

A. Amount of Monthly Income you need to support
your lifestyle @ $ _____
(*Debt payment, utilities, food, entertainment,
  education, etc.)

B. Current Investments which could be quickly converted
to cash @ $ _____ ÷ monthly income needed @ $ _____
= _____ months.

C. Income you expect from receivables if disabled *
which could go to support lifestyle: 1st month   @ _____
(i.e., after business expenses.)   2nd month @ _____
                                                  3rd month @ _____

Elimination Period Calculation =
# of months receivables will support you @ +   _____
# of months liquid investments support you @ +   _____
                                                               -- 3 (months)

= Elimination period in months @   _____
Income Needed Calculation:
Income needed to support your lifestyle @   _____

Less expected income from assets not used
in liquidity analysis such as Pension Plan
assets, I.R.A., Income partnerships —
multiply value of these assets by .005 =   _____

Amount of income you must get from disability
income insurance @ $ _____

Note: Benefit Period should always be at least to Age 65 for sickness or ac-
      cident, and usually lifetime for both sickness and accident.

Fig. 6-3. Simplified disability insurance worksheet.

Key contract provisions that you should have in your policy are in Table 6-2. In addition to the contract provisions listed, some other considerations you should explore are the possibility of having a "graded" or step premium policy that keeps your premiums low for a few years, gradually rising until they stay level after a set number of years. Graded premium policies are especially helpful for the younger physician who is getting started and needs a substantial amount of quality protection and has a limited budget. These policies are an excellent buy; however, they usually are only available to physicians under the age of forty.

For physicians who plan on having substantial salary increases and will be needing more disability insurance in the future, a policy with a future increase option benefit would allow you to purchase more disability income insurance regardless of your future health. Thus, if after you purchased your policy and became diabetic or had back problems, you could have your policy's benefit increased without any riders or waivers on your health problems.

When it comes to disability income insurance, expect to pay a healthy premium for the best coverage. It is much better to have a $2,000 a month policy that has very favorable contract provisions than to have a policy that will pay you $4,000 a month but has limitations and loopholes.

There is tremendous competition among insurance companies to get the physician's disability insurance business, and there are a number of very fine insurance companies out there providing favorable policies. If you have a disability policy today, it would be a good idea for you to mail your insurance company a letter to find out exactly how they would handle certain claims that you may incur. Figure 6-4 is a sample letter that you should mail to your insurance company. You should have it rewritten on your stationery and mail it out to your existing disability income insurance carrier.

Once disabled, you cannot increase your coverage to help keep pace with inflation. A "cost of living" rider, however, can be added to most policies to offset inflation. These riders are very important if you are not able to purchase enough base insurance coverage or if you live a very expensive lifestyle. Figure 6-5 illustrates the importance of a cost of living benefit, by showing how inflation will ruin your disability policy purchasing power.

In addition to having disability income insurance to protect you and your family from the loss of income that you provide and use for personal needs, you should consider having disability income insurance to cover your office expenses. This policy is sometimes called office overhead expense or capital account overhead expense. These policies pay those costs that are associated with keeping your practice going while you are disabled so that you could come back to a viable business after a disability of short duration, such as 1 or 2 years or less.

Table 6-2
Evaluating Your Disability Policy

Important Contract Provision	Benefit and Importance of Provision
1. Payment at Age 65 or Lifetime benefit, if possible.	Pays you at least to Age 65, to provide long term security.
2. Favorable definition of disability, i.e.: 2-1. Your occupation.	"Your Occupation" definition protects your ability to earn a living doing what you do now. This policy will pay you even if you work in another profession.
2-2. With Residual.	Residual benefit provides a benefit tied to either earnings lost or percent of time spent at occupation lost due to disability. A benefit based on earnings lost is far superior to time lost and should always be purchased. In fact, an "earnings lost" residual policy is better than a "your occupation" policy. Some policies pay full benefits even if you earn up to 49% of your pre-disability pay.
3. Cost of Living/Inflation Protection Benefit.	Post-Disability Benefits can increase with inflation, i.e., price increases. This provision is very important. Minimum increase you should purchase is 6% a year up to 3 times policy benefit, i.e., current benefit of $4,000. monthly could raise to $12,000. monthly maximum. Some policies increase benefits regardless of inflation rate.
4. Non-cancellable/guaranteed renewable coverage.	Policy cannot be changed by anyone except you. Premiums are guaranteed not to increase above premium stated in policy.
5. Subsequent Disability Reoccurrence Provision.	Waives a new elimination period if following a disability, you become disabled again from the same or another cause.
6. Earnings definition should include pension contributions and all bonuses.	Helps assure you will get residual benefit.
7. Pre-existing conditions covered if listed on policy application.	Some policies only cover sickness or accidents first "manifest" while policy is in force, i.e., if you had back problems in high school and no problems since, and you injured your back, company could deny claim stating you had problems prior to buying policy.

Note: Your Disability Income Insurance Policy is the most important insurance you can own. Make sure your policy fits your needs completely and has no loopholes.

Re: Policy #

Dear Sirs:

I have the following questions regarding my policy with your Company.

1. a. What is the *definition* of disability?
   b. My specialty is _____. If I were unable to perform my specialty, would I be disabled?
2. If I am only *partially disabled*, does it give me a benefit?
3. a. If I am *partially disabled* and *working half time*, does it give me a benefit? If so, how much and for how long?
   b. If I am partially disabled and *earn one-half* of what I earned prior to disability, what would my benefit be?
4. If I had a *heart attack* and was out of work for 1year and then came back to work but only worked half days, would you pay me? If so, how much and for how long?
5. If I were disabled through a *heart attack* for a period of 3 years and then went back to work full time, most of my clients would have found other professionals to handle their needs. Would you pay me (if I was able to work full time) a benefit while rebuilding my practice? If you would pay me a benefit, what would that benefit be and for how long?
6. Are my *premium rates guaranteed* never to go up?
7. Does this policy pay a *dividend*?
8. Is this policy *cancellable* by you?
9. Does this policy cover *conditions existing* prior to my taking out the policy?
10. Does my policy have any waivers on it? If so, why?
11. a. Can I change the elimination period on my policy?
    b. What is my current elimination period?
12. Is there a waiver of premium benefit on my policy?
13. If I were disabled and collected benefits for 6 months and then I went back to work for 6 months, and then became disabled again, would I have to satisfy a new elimination period?
14. Does this policy have a presumptive disability benefit that pays me if I lose my sight, hearing, etc., even if I continue to work?
15. a. What is my policy's benefit period?
    b. Can my policy's benefit period be changed to a lifetime sickness/lifetime accident benefit? If so, at what cost?
16. Does my policy have a cost of living benefit that raises my benefit as the Consumer Price Index rises? Can I add this benefit? If so, what will it cost?
17. I have lost my policy, would you please send me forms to request a duplicate policy?
18. When was the last premium paid on this policy? When is the next premium due? What will that next premium be?
19. I am a non-smoker—does your policy offer a non-smoker discount?
20. Is my policy a participating dividend paying policy? If so, what dividends do you project? (I understand that dividends are not guaranteed.)
21. I am now in a group practice, does your company have a group billing discount?
22. Who is the owner on this policy?
23. Who is the beneficiary?

Please send the above information to me *in writing* as soon as possible.

Thank you in advance for your prompt attention.   Sincerely,

Fig. 6-4. Disability income insurance letter to insurance company (type on your own stationery).

Dollars required in future years to equal $1,000. of current purchasing power
(assuming the following annual rates of inflation).

At the end of	4%	6%	8%	10%
5 years	$1,220.	$1,340.	$ 1,470.	$ 1,610.
10 years	$1,480.	$1,790.	$ 2,160.	$ 2,590.
15 years	$1,800.	$2,400.	$ 3,170	$ 4,171.
20 years	$2,190.	$3,200.	$ 4,660.	$ 6,730.
25 years	$2,680.	$4,290.	$ 6,850.	$10,830.
30 years	$3,250.	$5,750.	$10,060.	$17,450.

During a disability, compare the growth of a $3,150 monthly benefit over twenty
years at six percent compounded annually and a benefit with the six percent annual
growth.

Year Monthly	Monthly Benefit	Cumulative Benefits with 6% Compounded Annual Growth	Cumulative Benefits without 6% Compound Annual Growth
1	$3,150.	$ 37,800.	$ 37,800.
2	$3,339.	$ 77,868.	$ 75,600.
5	$3,976.	$ 213,060.	$189,000.
10	$5,321.	$ 498,180.	$378,000.
15	$7,121.	$ 879,744.	$567,000.
20	$9,530.	$1,390,392.	$756,000.

Fig. 6-5. Inflation effect on the purchasing power of disability insurance.

In deciding what overhead expense policy is best, use similar criteria as
with purchasing personal policies. You should buy enough coverage to
pay only the expenses of maintaining your office should you become disabled. For example, rather than having all five staff members, maybe you
will only need one or two key staff members to answer the phone, do billings, collect payments, and take care of your bills, monthly expenses, etc.
Some of the better office overhead expense policies cover some debt service associated with your business, in addition to the normal expenses
such as utilities, taxes, insurance payments, staff costs, telephone answering services, legal services, professional car expenses, stationery, postage,
and laundry.

Financial Privacy

7

Financial privacy and confidentiality about the specifics of your financial situation should be of importance to all physicians. Physicians' earnings on average are higher than most any other profession or occupation in the United States, which causes professionals to be targets for lawsuits, investment charlatans, briberies, and other schemes dreamed up by those that are not too honest. Financial privacy is not illegal and does not mean trying to hide anything from the government, etc., it merely means you should be able to control the information that is known about yourself.

There are many simple ways that can minimize the hassles that you receive because you are a physician and thus tagged as someone in a higher income bracket. There are also simple techniques that can make it so that you can control and not miss out on important opportunities because of misinformation about your financial situation that is desiminated. For example, I have been to lunches with physicians where the physician will see a colleague walk across the room and he will say, "See that guy over there—he needs a financial planner desperately; he doesn't run his finances well. I just heard from his banker that he had to go down to get a line of credit to pay off all of his credit cards because he was in financial hot water." Bankers have said to me, when clients are renegotiating their various loans, statements such as "Sutherland, I don't think it's appropriate right now to do anything with your client's loan package since I hear that he is considering getting a divorce" or "I hear his partner is thinking about retiring" and "he recently had a heart attack and may cut back on his hours or move away from the area." As you can see by the above examples, even nonfinancial information that gets out about yourself, whether true or not, can have an effect on your financial life. As a result of this, it is very important that you are conscious of telling your family, friends, and close associates that they are not to discuss anything specific about your situation with anyone. I am not saying be paranoid or secretive, I am merely saying that it is important that your close associates understand that conversations that they have with you about your personal situation are to be kept in confidence.

The first place to start with in keeping things confidential is with your staff. You should explain to them that anything about your personal situation and the way the practice is run and managed is to be strictly confidential. This also applies to information about your patients; such information should not be released to others without your permission.

It should be expected that when a staff person leaves your employment, whether on good, bad, or indifferent terms, that everything that they learned about your situation, your clientele, and the way you manage your practice is to be kept in strict confidence.

I know a man who decided to sue for malpractice only after a physician's nurse explained to him over the phone that the physician, her employer, had misdiagnosed his case. This doctor's blabbermouth nurse was probably not even aware that she was jeopardizing her boss's financial security. Had she been properly coached to protect the doctor, however, a malpractice attorney would have missed a contingency.

A few specific methods you should use to keep your home phone calls at a minimum from sharks calling from mailing lists, is to use your business address or a post office box for magazine subscriptions, newsletters, and addresses that you use on any business or legal forms, also, if at all possible, avoid putting M.D. or D.O. as part of your name in your address for subscriptions and using your first initials, rather than your first name, can help. For subscriptions to personal periodicals I suggest you have them come in your spouse's or children's name.

Credit cards should be issued with your initials and your last name and you should have credit card statements (even the personal ones) come to your office address or post office box. Leave M.D. or D.O. off your checks and credit cards and sign your name without the M.D. Your wife should not sign her name Mrs. John Smith, M.D., but rather Gloria Smith or Mrs. Maria Smith. The "JRJ, MD" license plate is a sure sign that some kid looking for drugs will find the contents of your briefcase sitting in the car to be of value.

In regard to the personal financial information that you have to disclose to businesses such as the bank, mortgage company, credit card companies, or professionals such as attorneys, accountants, financial planners, or insurance agents, you should have a discussion with each of these businesses or professionals about confidentiality and how their organizations retain the confidentiality about the specifics of your situation. You should ask point blank whether they have a policy about confidentiality.

I find that an unlisted phone number is a hassle and very inconvenient for my friends and family; however, we have gotten around getting phone calls at night by listing our personal phone in my wife's name. Naturally my name and office number is in the phone book. Clients and friends do have access to my home phone number, however, I give it to them.

If information gets out about yourself that you know is wrong and you know the source you should get the record straight. If a story gets out that is true and can harm you, make sure you give your side and the logic behind your actions. Reputations are very important in our society and you must do everything you can possibly do to protect it.

The suggestions in this chapter are suggestions that should cause little inconvenience to your personal situation and may just help avoid a few hassles for you.

The following are some sample letters that can be used as models for retaining financial confidentiality.

Letter to a bank whose loans have been paid off:

> Dear *Name of Bank Officer*:
>
> I have recently paid off the above numbered loans with your financial institution and would appreciate receiving copies of forms you have filed showing you no longer have a lien against my assets (i.e., U.C.C. cancellations, etc.).
>
> Sincerely,
>
> I Am Confidential

Letter to Professional Advisors:

> Dear *Name of Professional Advisor (i.e. CPA, Attorney, Financial Planner, Insurance Agent, Banker, etc.)*:
>
> It is very important to me that all documents, correspondence, and files relating to my situation be kept in the strictest confidence. I would appreciate it if you would go so far as to not even mention that I am a client even if someone asks you as to whether I am a client or not. I would appreciate it if you would say "that information about my clientele is confidential." This is nothing against your services or against your firm nor has there been anything happening in my relationship with you that has prompted this letter. It is just very important to me that all information that I share with professionals such as yourself be kept strictly confidential.
>
> Sincerely yours,
>
> I Am Confidential

Letter to Health and Disability Insurance Agent:

> Dear *Insurance Agent*:
>
> On all documents where it is not necessary to list MD (or DO), please have these initials dropped from the end of my name.

Do not address me on these policies as Doctor, and please mail me the necessary forms to make it so that your policy records reflect just my first, middle name, and last name.

Sincerely,

I Am Confidential

Additional Steps To Financial Confidentiality:

1. Make all sensitive purchases with bank money orders or cash—keep a receipt for tax purposes.
2. Use "D.B.A." assumed name filings for large transactions or simple businesses that you get involved in. For example, own your office building under a D.B.A. such as "Main Street Investments."
3. Use cash for nondeductible expenses—avoid using your "Gold Card" for small purchases.
4. Take your name off your mail box, put your initials only. So friends can find you, paint a red square on the box.
5. Use a safety deposit box for some of your wealth. Own the box in a D.B.A., trust, or corporation. Photocopy the contents and keep a list of assets in the box.
6. Only deal with companies who have a reputation for a high degree of integrity, who you have checked out completely, i.e., references and check out financial stability of company and principals.
7. Check your credit records at local credit bureaus to assure that information is accurate.
8. Be honest with your records or don't disclose—Be aggressive in tax planning, but don't cheat—avoid audit.
9. Pay your bills on time and always have integrity in all business dealings.

RECOMMENDED READING

Mark Skousen's Complete Guide to Financial Privacy (1979)
Alexandria House
901 N. Washington Street
Alexandria, VA 22314

8

Use of Business Form to Maximize Wealth Creation

For physicians the proper use of business form can be a useful tool in minimizing risks, creating wealth, and reducing taxes. Utilization of a proper business form is one of the most important decisions a physician can make.

Up until about 30 years ago, a physician basically had 2 choices, either he could be a proprietorship, i.e., a solo practice, or a partnership. Thus, the choice of business form was not decided for tax reasons, but rather for practice or lifestyle reasons. In 1954, however, the United States Circuit Court of Appeals in the Kinter Clinic Case moved that it was okay for a group of incorporated physicians to adopt a pension plan and thus be treated as a professional corporation.

Up until that time professionals could not shelter income from their practices from taxes, deduct substantial retirement plan contributions, have medical reimbursement programs, favorable tax treatment on life and disability insurance, etc. Even when the Keogh plans were allowed in 1962, if you were an unincorporated business, you could only deduct up to $1,250 per year for retirement. So for a high earning physician, a corporation was the answer. Today over half of the physicians who are not working for major corporations or hospitals are incorporated. Today the latest Tax Acts have made it so that regardless of whether you are a corporation, a proprietorship, or partnership, you can have a retirement plan virtually identical to what only a few years ago was available only to a professional corporation.

Even though there is now parity in retirement plans, however, there are many other advantages to corporations. Table 8-1 shows the advantages and disadvantages of the four primary types of business forms you may choose, i.e., proprietorship, partnership, solo corporations, or a corporation with two or more physicians practicing.

A proprietorship is the most simple form of business ownership. A proprietorship does not protect you from liability and it does not allow you to shift income as you may be able to do in a corporate business form. A proprietorship is the easiest business to start and is the least expensive to operate.

Table 8-1
Business Form Comparison

	Proprietor-ship	Partnership	Solo Corporation	Two or more doctor Corporation
Limits liability	No	No	Yes—not for malpractice	Yes—not for personal malpractice
Ability to shift income	No	Very limited	Yes—with old P.C.'s No—with new P.C.'s	Yes—with old P.C.'s No—with new P.C.'s
Reduces taxes on excess income not needed for lifestyle, i.e., use of two tax brackets	No	No	Yes	Yes
Ease of bringing in new associates	Becomes partnership	Some	Easy	Easier and becomes easier as more associates brought into corporation
Ease of operation	Easiest	Slightly easier than two-doctor corporation	More complicated than proprietorship	Most complicated, however, not much more than partnership
Expenses of operation	Lowest cost	Slightly less than corporation	About same as as partnership, more than proprietorship	Cost per physician goes down as more doctors in practice
Fringe Benefits:				
Tax Favored Retirement Plans				
Loans to physicians/owners	No	No	Yes	Yes
Benefit and contribution limits	Same	Same	Same	Same
Tax favored disability plan	No	No	Yes	Yes
Tax favored purchase of life insurance				
through pension plan	Yes	Yes	Yes	Yes
through group insurance	No	No	Yes	Yes
through "split dollar" plan	No	No	Yes	Yes
Tax favored discriminatory deferred compensation plan (in excess of pension plan benefits	No	No	Yes	Yes—works excellent in large P.C.'s
Tax favored medical/dental program	No	No	Yes	Yes
Estate Planning				
Ease of practice continuation at death, disability, retirement	Practice stops unless special Buy/Sell set up	Partnership must be reorganized. Should have Buy/Sell Agreement	Practice stops unless special Buy/Sell Agreement has been drawn.	Should have Buy/Sell Employment contract; if corporation does, is very easy

Note: Seek competent professional help prior to forming a corporation or deciding on proper business forms. Only incorporate if it makes sense.

From Financial & Investment Planning, Ltd., Suttons, Bay, MI. With permission.

However, after factoring in taxes when comparing a proprietorship to a corporation, often a proprietorship can be a more expensive form than a corporation, even though the legal and accounting costs of incorporating are an added expense. A partnership is in many ways similar to proprietorships in that it does not help much in tax planning, nor does it offer any tax-favored fringe benefit programs. Partnerships can, however, create some special legal technicalities that must be considered. In a partnership you may be liable for mistakes and liabilities of your partner, while a corporation can help shield you from your associates' legal liabilities.

In a professional corporation you used to be able to stagger your corporate year to something different than a calendar year and thus throw income into the next year. In addition, the corporation is a separate entity and thus has its own tax and legal status. A corporation pays taxes at a rate that can be very conducive to creating wealth for its owners.

While a corporation has some substantial benefits, there are also some negatives to incorporating. Primarily, you will have greater legal and accounting costs. In some states you may have to pay premiums for disability insurance to the state in addition to unemployment insurance, and you may have to be covered under workers' compensation laws.

The primary advantage of an incorporated form of business is: In a tax-favored retirement plan you could have loans to the physicians/owners in the program up to $50,000 while if you were an unincorporated physician you could not. The corporation can provide tax-favored life insurance benefits through the purchase of a group life insurance whereby you can deduct up to the cost of purchasing $50,000 term insurance.

Any life insurance group plan must be nondiscriminatory, i.e., must cover other employees in your practice, and the plan must be in writing. While this benefit may seem substantial, most physicians will find that it is cheaper to purchase their life insurance through some other method since covering the employees for such a small amount of life insurance can be very expensive. Also because insurance is cheaper per thousand, when bought in large quantities, it is often very expensive to purchase a $50,000 policy when compared to purchasing a policy of a substantially greater death benefit, perhaps in a different method such as: (1) purchasing of your insurance through your pension plan, or (2) purchasing your insurance on a corporate split dollar basis. Both of these plans let you use a favorable tax status of another entity to reduce the after tax cost of providing your family with this valuable benefit.

If you purchase your life insurance through your pension plan, this allows you to substantially deduct your premium. You have to pay taxes only on the pure insurance costs associated with the purchase of life insurance through your pension plan. Chapter 16 on retirement planning will deal with this in greater detail. A very popular benefit of a corporation is the providing of a split dollar insurance through the corporation often in tandem with a deferred compensation agreement.

A split dollar program or the purchasing of life insurance through your corporate retirement plan can be done on a discriminatory basis. This allows you to free-up those dollars that you may be paying to insurance on a personal basis so they could go to other lifestyle needs or to create wealth for yourself while saving taxes along the way. A corporation allows you to deduct your disability income insurance premium and thus makes your disability policy substantially tax-favored. If your corporation does deduct your disability insurance, all benefits coming from your disability insurance will come to you taxable. You can, however, use what is called split dollar disability insurance program, whereby part of your disability program will come to you tax-free and part on a taxable basis.

Many insurance salesmen are unfamiliar with this technique so you might bring it up at your annual insurance review.

Dr. I. M. Sample (Table 8-2) is an illustration of the utilization of a corporate business form over being a sole practitioner. This example shows how the corporation is taxed at a much lower rate on extra earnings than an individual can be. On those extra earnings you should be able to presently accumulate up to $150,000 without any questions from the I.R.S. However, check with your tax advisor on this prior to accumulating $150,000. You can accumulate a greater amount than that if you are considering expanding your practice or may want to buy buildings in the future or if your practice is substantial and you could justify the need of having more than $150,000. You could set up a salary continuation or deferred compensation program with these excess earnings and they could accumulate substantially tax-free.

Another advantage of accumulating wealth on a corporate basis is that you could purchase high yielding dividend paying preferred and common stocks and have these dividends 80 percent tax free in your corporation. This could help you build wealth efficiently. An added point for financial planning—your liquidity should be in your corporation. You should not pay out a large salary to yourself to build up your personal liquidity. You should keep your liquidity and your liquid cash in the corporation, as this is the most tax-favored place to keep it, especially if it is invested in high yielding common stocks. If you ever have a financial trauma such as a disability or a family problem that requires some cash, you can always draw out of your corporation at that time. All the while this money is accumulating on a tax-favored basis.

Through the corporate form it is much easier to transfer your practice than it would be with as a sole proprietorship or as a partnership format. Once you have a set formula for selling your stock in your corporation at death, disability, or retirement, etc., you do not have to keep redrawing and redrafting documentation each time a partner comes or goes. It is already in writing and it is just the execution of that document format if somebody wishes to leave your practice or come into the practice. This also helps with your personal estate planning.

Table 8-2.
Simplified Sample Comparison of Corporate or
Proprietorship Business Forms.

Dr. I. AM. SAMPLE
Income to Lifestyle and Wealth Creation at $100,000

Non/corporate form		Corporation
$ 48,000.	Income needed for lifestyle after taxes	$ 48,000.
$ 11,000.	Approximate taxes on income	$ 11,000.
$ 1,000.	Approximate accounting and legal costs	$ 1,800.
$ 2,000.	Disability insurance premium	$ 2,000.
$ 600.*	+ Tax cost	$ 0.*
$ 10,000.	Profit sharing and pension deposit	$ 10,000.
$ 550.	Cost to maintain plans	$ 550.
$ 1,500.	Health insurance plan	$ 1,500.
$ 550. *	+ Tax cost	$ 0.*
$ 75,000.	Totals	$ 74,850.
$ 24,800.	Amount left to go towards . . . . wealth creation	$ 25,150.
	Less corporate tax . . . . $	3,775.
-$ 7,000.	Less personal tax Amount left to use to create wealth	
$ 17,800.	for physician	$ 21,375.

* Proper deductible.

Notes: You should have your accountant, tax attorney, or planning specialist run the numbers similar to the above prior to incoporating your practice. The above is over-simplified and even if your situation is similar to our sample, you must factor in unemployment insurance, workers' compensation costs, etc., if applicable in your state. Also, legal and accounting costs vary from state to state. This chart should not be considered legal or accounting advice.

From Financial & Investment Planning, Ltd., Suttons Bay, MI. With permission.

Another primary advantage of incorporating is that it can help protect you from the liabilities of the other physicians in your practice. Each state is different in liability laws and liability laws regarding this are complicated. Your attorney can brief you in greater detail on the advantages of incorporating to protect yourself against the liabilities of the other physicians in your practice.

Before deciding to incorporate, you must sit down with your advisors and go through an exercise similar to the exercise illustrated in Table 8-1. The example is oversimplified; however, it does show the chronology of deciding whether to incorporate. There are other methodologies for this decision-making process and your tax attorney, accountant, or financial planning professional can help you run the numbers on your own practice. Remember it is easy to incorporate; however, it is expensive to unincorporate. So make sure before you incorporate that it will be to your advantage and make sure that your advisors are knowledgeable about the utilization of pension and profit sharing plans and other fringe benefit programs in corporations.

Buy Your Kids an Ice Cream Store

9

From my experience, the anxiety that physicians feel about accumulating wealth for educating their children is greater than the anxiety that they feel toward accumulating wealth for their own financial security and retirement. Where this malaise came from does not matter, but the reality of the situation is that for most physicians after providing their family with financial security through a properly proportioned risk management program, educating their children is the next priority.

It is true that college costs can run into an excess of $15,000 per year and that with inflation these costs could double or triple in the next 10–20 years. With physicians' incomes leveling out and not keeping pace with inflation, many physicians are having tremendous anxiety about educating their children. First of all, do not worry. It is not your responsibility to pay for your children's college costs. No one makes you do it—you choose to pay for their costs. Many parents choose not to pay for their children's college costs and somehow their children still seem to make it through college with good grades and without a lot of discomfort. Statistics show that over 50 percent of children's college education costs are not paid for by their parents. In fact, many parents pay none and by some statistical evidence only 14 percent of parents pay most of their children's college education costs. I have formulated three postulates regarding educating children from my experience as a financial planner for physicians. They are: (1) Do not give the money to the child unless they earn it, (2) Make the money that goes toward the child's college education tax deductible, and (3) You should retain 100 percent control of any money that did not go to the child by methods number 1 and 2, i.e., keep the money in your name and under your control.

I had a client who over the years had put $20,000 into his child's name under Uniform Gift to Minors Act. As soon as the child turned 18 she found out about the $20,000 and flew to Southern California and her parents have not heard from her since. I always wondered what would have happened if her parents had not put the money in her name and kept it in their own name and said to their child when she turned 18, "Over the years we set aside a little nest egg to pay for your college costs should you wish to to go. If you would like to go to college, we will pay the freight." Knowing both the parents and the child, I know that with the encouragement of having the college costs paid for, the child would have gone to college. However, when the child realized that she had $20,000 in cash, she decided it would be more fun to live it up for a few years.

Another reason that I do not recommend putting money in children's names is that if sizeable sums are transferred to your child's name, the end result could be to reduce the financial aid granted to your child when they apply for grants and scholarships. In some cases schools would expect much less of a contribution from the family if the money had just been left in the parents' names instead of having put it in the child's name. It must be understood that on paper the "popular" methods of transferring wealth to your children may sound great; however, in practice they do not work. Table 9-1 lists some of the methods of creating wealth for your child's college education costs. My number one postulate is do not give the money to the child unless they earn it. The best way to pay for college costs is with tax deductible dollars. The only way to pay for children's college costs with tax deductible dollars is to hire them to work for you or your professional corporation. This makes all the costs, every dollar you pay them, tax deductible at the child's lower tax bracket. The money that goes to your child must be reasonable for the duties that they perform. You cannot pay them $15.00 per hour for an $8.00 per hour job. Also, your children must legitimately show up to work and perform the duties that they are paid for, be they cleaning the office, doing your computerized billings, filing, being a "go-for," washing your business auto, etc. The Tax Reform Act 1986 made putting your child on salary more complicated. Consult your tax advisor on this technique.

Hiring your child to work for you is a tried and true method of allowing you to transfer tax deductible wealth to your child. If you are in the 32 percent tax bracket and you transfer a dollar to yourself and then pay what is left to your child, your child is going to end up with 68 cents on the dollar going toward college education costs. While if it is deductible through your corporation or your business, your child is going to end up with 85–90 cents on the dollar.

If you work for a hospital or are in corporate practice where all your other partners and colleagues are doing the same thing, it would not be practical to hire your child, but buy them an ice cream store and put them into business for themselves. Being in business for themselves (as your partner) will be a better education, perhaps even better than they will get at college. It also makes their college costs deductible. Do not worry about the business losing money because of your child's salary. It can lose money for a few years. Who knows, maybe your child's business will become the next Haagen Daz's or Orville Redenbacker. If you like the idea of putting your child into business for themselves, try to put them into a business that has low start up costs. There are a number of books out that discuss the many options available for starting up businesses at a low cost. You should sit down with your child and discuss the different options and decide which option you both feel the most comfortable with.

Table 9-1
Creating Wealth For College Costs

Method	Advantages	Disadvantages
Hire them to work for you or your P.C.	Makes costs deductible; child earns his/her way through college.	Disruption of staff. Child's pay must be legitimate and reasonable.
Put them into business (buy them an ice cream store)	Expenses are deductible; such as child's wages. Gives child "hands-on" experience and responsibility. Child earns way through college.	Costs of setting up business. Child may enjoy being in business so much he/she may quit college to be full-time.
Have child work for someone else.	Child will learn to work hard and have self-confidence because he/she did it substantially on their own.	
Sale or gift and lease-back	Helps make college costs deductible; makes depreciated assests generate additional tax savings.	Once money is put into child's name, it is theirs; make sure you get competent help in setting up this method.
Use personal funds, sell the stock, cash in the municpial bond, call in that loan to your brother-in-law, cash in or borrow on that old insurance policy.	Simplest method. Let's you keep control of the money, which can, hopefully, then be paid out in one of the methods above when child goes to college.	If you do not pay money out by method as above, then costs are not deductible; this is an expensive method.
Borrow from your P.C.	If the P.C. has the cash, take it and pay it back over time.	Make sure you have your attorney or accountant advise you on how to set this up.
Borrow it from your bank, parents, credit union, etc. If the bank, parents, credit union say "No," borrow from your retirement plans.	Allows your retirement plans to stay intact; if you have trouble paying it back, draw on your retirement plans.	Only do this if you have created a lot of wealth already in your retirement plans; don't jeopardize your own financial security for your child's education.
Uniform Gift to Minor's Act (U.G.M.A.)	Interest and dividend earnings on the U.G.M.A. account are taxable in the child's tax bracket if over age 14 or under $500.00 in earnings. (When you compare the alternatives, U.G.M.A.'s etc., are a bad deal.)	Once deposited, it is your child's money and at the age of majority they can do whatever they want with the money. The deposits to the U.G.M.A. are not deductible.

Note: The above should not be considered legal or accounting advice. A combination of the above methods works best.

From Financial & Investment Planning, Ltd., Suttons, Bay, MI. With permission.

If you own any rental properties, perhaps you should have your child start a property maintenance and management company and he or she can be in charge of maintaining your property, renting it out, taking care of the maintenance lease details, and perhaps do it for a few of your friends and colleagues.

In addition to hiring your child or putting them into business for themselves, there is nothing wrong with having your child go to work for someone else. There are dozens of people who have waited tables, worked as a night janitor, lifeguarded, short order cook, or busperson to get through college. In addition to providing much needed funds for your child's education, the money that your child is able to earn on their own will make them feel confident and will teach him or her the importance of the work ethic. Working their way through college will help increase your child's self-confidence and teach her or him to get along with other people. Colleges do not teach us people skills; however, working in the real world forces you to learn good communication, people skills, and responsibility.

Another popular method of earning college costs is to take your depreciated assets, either sell them or gift them to your child or to a trust for the child as the beneficiary, and then have your practice lease them back from the trust or your child. These dollars, which are completely deductible to you, can go to help pay for the child's college education costs. Before doing a sale or gift and lease back program, it is very important that you seek competent professional help in the methodologies of setting up such a program. Your accountant or corporate tax attorney should be familiar with this methodology. Ideally, your child should be over 14 if you use this technique and thus avoid having the income taxed at your bracket (rather than the child's).

The most simple method to pay for your child's college education costs is to take your personal funds and use that money to pay for the college costs, be it selling your 100 shares of IBM or cashing in your local hospital bonds. This method allows you to keep control of your assets and then you can utilize those assets as you wish to help pay for your child's college education costs. The problem with this method is that you are not paying for your child's college education costs with tax deductible dollars. Also, the earnings on your assets, if they are assets that throw off a lot of taxable earnings, will be taxable at your higher tax bracket.

If you or your PC do not have a lot of money, the next place to find the money is to borrow it from your bank, credit union, parents, etc. This allows you to get the much needed cash for your child's education. You are, however, sacrificing some of your financial future if you utilize this method without having a substantial amount of wealth built up in your IRAs or retirement plans. If you have a substantial amount of wealth created in your retirement plans or IRAs, there is nothing wrong with borrowing to pay college costs off over a great number of years, rather than borrowing or cashing in your retirement plans.

Table 9-2 shows how even if you were to cash in your IRA or pension plan after a number of years, you could still come out ahead over not having funded your pension plan because of the tax deferred growth of the retirement plan. If you do not have the ability to borrow money from the bank or if you do not feel comfortable borrowing the money and you do have a substantial amount of money in your retirement plan, there is nothing wrong with cashing in one of your IRAs or borrowing from your pension plan to pay for your child's college education costs.

The following methods of creating wealth for college education costs are methods that are like playing with dynamite and should only be used because none of the aforementioned methods will fit your situation. These methods basically take your money and transfer the money into an Uniform Gift to Minors Act Account. The primary disadvantage of these methods is that deposits made to these accounts are not currently tax deductible. And if your child is under 14 you will have the money taxed back in your tax bracket. Only the earnings from these accounts grow at a lower bracket and when you consider that you could purchase tax-free municipal bonds, variable or fixed annuities, real estate limited partnerships, or leasing partnerships that throw off tax-sheltered income, and other techniques to reduce the income generated from assets, the transfer of these assets to children becomes impotent.

Table 9-2
Example of Value of Tax Deferral; Assuming I.R.A.
Early Withdrawal 10% Penalty

| | Pension or I.R.A. Breakeven Holding Periods | | | | | | | | | | |
| | Average annual yield to withdrawal* | | | | | | | | | | |

Constant Marginal Tax Rate * (%)	6%	7%	8%	9%	10%	11%	12%	13%	14%	15%	16%	17%
10	19.63	16.83	14.72	13.09	11.78	10.71	9.82	9.06	8.41	7.85	7.36	6.93
15	13.91	11.92	10.43	9.27	8.34	7.59	6.95	6.42	5.96	5.56	5.22	4.91
20	11.13	9.54	8.35	7.42	6.68	6.07	5.56	5.14	4.77	4.45	4.17	3.93
25	9.54	8.18	7.16	6.36	5.72	5.20	4.77	4.40	4.09	3.82	3.58	3.37
30	8.56	7.34	6.42	5.71	5.14	4.67	4.28	3.95	3.67	3.43	3.21	3.02
35	7.96	6.82	5.97	5.30	4.77	4.34	3.98	3.67	3.41	3.18	2.98	2.81
40	7.60	6.51	5.70	5.06	4.56	4.14	3.80	3.51	3.26	3.04	2.85	2.68
45	7.43	6.37	5.57	4.95	4.46	4.05	3.72	3.43	3.19	2.97	2.79	2.62
50	7.44	6.38	5.58	4.69	4.46	4.06	3.72	3.43	3.19	2.98	2.79	2.63

*Rates are continuously compounded for both taxes and average annual yield. Rates not continuously compounded can be substituted for a rough idea of the breakeven point. Example: If you are in a 30% tax bracket and you earn 12% on your I.R.A., in 4.28 years you will be at "breakeven." This means that even if you cashed in your I.R.A. and paid a 10% penalty plus current income taxes on your withdrawal, you would be ahead if you did it after 4.28 years (over not having had an I.R.A.).

In some special situations and cases these methods can work, i.e., a child over 14. However, make sure you work with a competent financial planning professional who knows how to utilize the other methods and is extremely competent in working with these methods of transferring wealth.

The Uniform Gift to Minors Act (UGMA). Under the UGMA, the money is placed in your child's name with you, your spouse, grandparent, or whomever as a custodian, and your job as custodian is to invest those assets in a manner that will allow those assets to grow for your child. You are basically a fiduciary and your job is to oversee those assets. Once those assets are put into a UGMA account, that money is your child's and will revert to your child when he or she reaches the age of majority. You cannot transfer the money back to your account and the deposits you make to the UGMA account are not deductible; only the earnings in the account grow, tax deferred, as they are taxed at your child's lower tax bracket, if your child is over age 14 or earns under $500.

As mentioned in my three postulates, you lose control over that money as soon as your child reaches the age of majority, so he or she could fly to Hawaii, buy a new Porsche, or give it to that new church in town.

As previously stated, there is nothing wrong with borrowing or cashing in part of your retirement plan trust to pay for your child's education costs. In fact, this method can be the most cost-effective method when compared to the Uniform Gift to Minors Act, etc. In educating your children you will most likely use a number of the methods illustrated in this chapter.

If your child decides to go to a $15,000-a-year college, it is going to be very hard for him or her to make enough money working or being in business for himself or herself, during the 3-month college summer break, the Christmas and Easter breaks, etc., so you are going to have to come up with money from other methods. These methods will also work to pay for precollege, private high schools, vocational training, or other special training that your child may desire, such as learning a foreign language in another country or going on an educational trip to remote islands to study turtles.

ADDRESSES

To get your children's social security numbers, visit your local Social Security Office or write:

Social Security Administration
P.O. Box 57
Baltimore, Maryland 21203

To get your Statement of Earnings from Social Security Administration, write to the above and ask for it, over your signature. (You should do this every 2–3 years.)

10

Investment Strategies—Understanding Our Cyclical Economy

Our economy is cyclical because people are cyclical. We go from periods of extreme optimism to a pessimism that makes us store up food, buy guns, and move to the country. These swings in the mass psychology of people are what move our investment markets. This psychology, which will be reflected in our financial markets, comes from peoples' reactions to the current and perceived financial state of affairs.

Understanding the four basic cycles that will happen in our economy and financial markets can help you to create wealth for yourself no matter what the market.

MONEY CAN BE MADE IN ANY ECONOMIC CYCLE

Any decision involving money or assets over time is an investment decision. Thus, it is very important that you analyze the cycle that we are in, the cycle that we are coming from, and the cycle that we are moving toward on a continuous basis in order to stay on top of protecting your wealth and making it grow.

The most positive of these cycles is the *Wealth Creation Economy*. In a wealth creation economy there is real economic growth, generally low inflation, and stability in prices. There is low unemployment and some growth in the labor force, productivity growth, and, very importantly, advances in technology and innovation. In fact the brilliant economist Joseph Schumpeler vividly illustrated how innovation and technological changes supplied favorable cyclical economic force.

The years 1950–1969 were characterized as a wealth creation economy. During that time the best investments were in businesses of the kind that grew and prospered during this period. A well-run, well-managed business will do the best in a wealth creation economy. Thus, common stocks, limited partnerships, and investments representing ownership of businesses did extremely well during this period. Also during this period real estate in many areas of the country created a tremendous capital gain for its owners. Table 11-1 (see page 88) illustrates basically the period from 1966–1985 in graphic form showing the real economic growth, inflation rate, unemployment rate, stock market performance, changes in the price of gold, and productivity gains for that period. The two periods of a wealth creation economy, 1950–1969, and 1983–1987, are highlighted as a wealth creation economy.

The second part of the economic cycle is the *Wealth Transfer Economy*. The characteristics of a wealth Transfer Economy are high inflation and prices increasing faster than wages. There is often high unemployment in the private sector and poor productivity for those that are working. The period from 1971–1979 will give you an illustration of this type of economy. In this type of economy, normal financial morals become topsy-turvy. During a Wealth Transfer Economy, placing your investment assets in investments such as savings accounts, bonds, money market instruments, CDs, most common stocks, etc., can be disastrous. Even if your CD returns you 10 percent, if inflation is at 10 percent, you have just broken even on your money, and because that 10 percent interest you earned on your CD could be fully taxable, your returns are reduced further.

The best investments during this period are tangible investments such as gold, silver, precious metals, well-selected (1) collectibles, (2) common stocks, (3) real estate, and investments in countries that are in a stable wealth creation economic cycle. For example, Swiss investments performed very favorably in the 1970s.

The next economic cycle, which can be characterized by the Great Depression, is the *Wealth Destruction Economy*. Hallmarks of a Wealth Destruction Economy are high unemployment and low productivity, falling prices, negative growth, and a feeling of pessimism among individuals. The best investments to own just before and during the Wealth Destruction Economy are U.S. Government Bonds and bonds of the highest grades, FDIC and FSLIC insured CDs and high yielding common stocks in industries with a near monopoly, such as utilities, some energy companies, etc.

The sister of the Wealth Destruction Economy would be the *Crisis Economy* and the chances of having a Crisis Economy in our lifetimes are probably greater than the chances of having a Wealth Destruction Economy.

A Crisis Economy is characterized by high unemployment and torrid inflation rates (such as what was experienced in Argentina, 415 percent). In the Crisis Economy, wages are rising much slower than prices. There is low productivity. There is negativism about the future and a great disparity often develops between the wealthy and the poor in the society at the expense of the middle class. This causes political and social unrest and can lead to crisis, as has happened in many countries in South America and Africa in the last few decades (this also happened in Europe hundreds of years ago).

The best strategy during the crisis cycle is to first move your investments to another country that is in a stable Wealth Creation Economy, or to move your family to another country if the crisis becomes acute. During a Crisis Economy it is important to be nimble and quick with your investments. The most important thing during a cycle like this is to stay liquid and to balance your investments between tangibles such as gold and silver, treasury bills, high grade money market instruments, and short-term CDs, while avoiding rare stuff such as rare coins, stamps, etc., and common stocks and long-term bonds.

It also makes sense during a Crisis Economy to stock up on food, fuel, and paper products. If the cycle happens to be in the United States, it is extremely important to analyze whether you feel that the U.S. will move out of the Crisis Economy and if so to "bottom fish" for investments because people that make proper investments during the Crisis Economy will become the millionaires of tomorrow. The investments to bottom fish for will be long-term extremely high yielding government bonds or high grade corporate bonds, and as interest rates start falling and bonds rally, and things look slightly hopeful, move your money to diversified portfolios of well selected common stocks, buying the stocks with both feet.

In all of the economic cycles mentioned, it makes sense to do bottom fishing. In the cycle of the Wealth Creation Economy, if you start seeing economic growth slow down, the inflation rate moving up, and the unemployment rate rising slightly, it would make sense to sell those investments that made you money during that cycle and invest your money in Treasury Bills, bonds, or money market instruments until you can decide what the next economy we will be moving into will be and then purchase investments that will perform the best during the next economic cycle. Tremendous wealth will be created by those individuals that are confidently able to buy the investments against the grain of mass psychology before the next cycle and sell as we move fully into the next economic cycle. An outline of the individual basic economic cycles can be found on the pages that follow.

This book cannot tell you what to do, but will show you how to formulate a plan of action to help you make investment decisions that will help you prosper during the economic and business cycles. Chapter 12 will deal with specific investment forms and how to analyze whether a specific investment form is reasonably priced so that you can make better investment choices after you decide what economic cycle we are in. The first decision of investment is to figure out what investment cycle we are in and then to decide which investments seem under-valued in relationship to this cycle and the next.

ECONOMIC CYCLES—CRISIS ECONOMY

CHARACTERISTICS:

- High unemployment
- Torrid inflation
- Wages rising must slower than prices
- Low productivity
- High taxes, citizen unrest
- Great disparity developing between wealthy and poor, with middle class becoming a minority

BEST INVESTMENTS:

- Move to another country
- Balance investments between tangibles such as gold and silver (not rare stuff), T-bills, money market instruments, FSLIC or FDIC insured CDs, investments in wealth creation economies (other countries)
- Stock up on food, fuel, paper products and stay liquid to bottom fish

BOTTOM FISH INVESTMENTS:

- When interest rates seem out of this world, buy long term government bonds, or highest grade corporate bonds—after bond rally, buy common stocks with both feet.

WEALTH DESTRUCTION ECONOMY

CHARACTERISTICS:

- Falling prices
- Negative growth
- High unemployment
- High rate of business failures
- Few new businesses started

ECONOMIC CYCLES—WEALTH TRANSFER ECONOMY

CHARACTERISTICS:

- High inflation/prices increasing faster than wages
- High unemployment, poor productivity
- Negative real economic growth
- High taxes on earnings

BEST INVESTMENTS:

- Tangible investments (gold, silver, etc.), well selected real estate, well selected common stocks, investments in countries in a wealth creation economy

11

Investment Strategies—Only One Investment Goal

There should be only one investment goal—high total returns."Growth," "income," "capital gains," and other investment goals must be discarded because what every investor wants is one dollar to grow to two dollars, and then to three dollars, and so on. Whether that total return comes from growth, income, or capital gains, the result is the same. You are now saying, but what about taxes and what about inflation? Taxes and inflation both will affect the total returns on your investment. You must not, however, make your investment decisions based completely on taxes and on inflation. Naturally, if your are in a high tax bracket, it makes more sense to have your returns come from a tax-favored methodology than from a taxable one. If you could earn twice as much money in a taxable situation than you can in a tax-favored one, it would probably be smarter to go with the taxable method. Too many individuals make their decisions based purely on taxes or purely on "buzzwords" such as "I want growth, capital gains, etc." The primary decision is to have "real returns," real total returns after inflation and taxes.

You learned in Chapter 10 that our economy is cyclical and that while certain growth investments may be better during some economic cycles than during others, you do not want to buy into the philosophy that all you want is growth investments during the cycle where growth investments would not perform favorably. Nor do you want or need an investment such as a Treasury bill, bond, or money market instrument that may be great during an economic cycle such as a Wealth Destruction Economy while being a very mediocre performer during a Wealth Creation Economy where your growth common stocks and real estate investments should perform very favorably.

Table 11-1 shows how to figure the total return on CDs, bonds, or most growth and income investments. Note that this figure illustrates the impact of taxes and inflation on your investment. It also figures the total return after taxes and inflation. If you can have a total return after taxes and inflation of 3-6 percent, you should feel happy with your investment

Table 11-1
Annual Total Return of Assets

Year	Growth Rate of Real GNP	Inflation Rate all Items	Unemployment All Workers	Productivity Output per 1 Paid Hour	U.S. Federal Budget as % of GNP	Gold	U.S. Common Stocks	U.S. Government Bonds	U.S. Business Real Estate	International Stocks E,A,FE	Cycle
'66	2.7%	2.9%		1960 @ 65.2%	0.5%		-8.21%	4.08%	4.00%		Wealth Creation
'67	4.6%	2.9%		1965 @ 78.4%	1.1%		30.45%	-4.49%	6.39%		Wealth Creation
'68	2.8%	4.2%			3.0%	@ 12.29%	14.95%	1.93%	10.69%		Wealth Creation
'69	-0.2%	5.4%	3.5%		surplus	@ 5.60%	-9.86%	-2.82%	6.09%		Wealth Creation
'70	3.4%	5.9%	4.9%	86.2%	0.3%	@ 12.29%	-1.00%	14.58%	9.99%	-14.10%	Wealth Creation
'71	5.7%	4.3%	5.9%		2.2%	@ 13.19%	18.16%	9.75%	15.49%	26.10%	Wealth Creation
'72	5.8%	3.3%	5.6%		2.1%	@ 42.13%	17.71%	4.82%	9.49%	33.30%	Oil Crisis
											(Wealth Transfer)
'73	-0.6%	6.2%	4.9%		1.2%	48.00%	-18.68%	2.03%	7.39%	-16.80%	Wealth Transfer
'74	-1.2%	11.0%	5.6%	94.5%	.0%	66.00%	-27.77%	8.23%	8.09%	-25.60%	Wealth Transfer
'75	5.4%	9.1%	8.6%		3.1%	-24.00%	37.49%	7.82%	8.86%	31.20%	Wealth Transfer
'76	5.5%	5.8%	8.5%		4.0%	-4.00%	26.68%	12.73%	8.02%	-0.40%	Wealth Creation
'77	5.0%	6.5%	7.1%		2.4%	22.50%	3.03%	2.00%	8.99%	14.60%	Wealth Creation
'78	2.8%	7.7%	6.1%	100.6%	2.3%	37.00%	8.53%	2.05%	12.17%	28.90%	Wealth Transfer
'79	-0.3%	11.3%	5.8%	99.4%	1.2%	131.90%	24.18%	4.42%	14.52%	1.80%	Wealth Transfer
'80	2.5%	13.5%	7.1%	99.0%	2.8%	12.50%	33.22%	3.38%	11.42%	19.00%	Wealth Transfer
'81	-2.1%	10.4%	7.6%	101.3%	2.6%	-32.20%	-5.00%	-1.00%	9.8%	-4.90%	Crisis
											(Transfer Year)
'82	2.5%	6.1%	9.7%	101.2%	4.1%	-14.20%	21.60%	40.00%	13.30%	-4.60%	Wealth Creation
'83	3.6%	3.2%	9.6%	103.9%	6.3%	-16.50%	22.60%	5.80%	9.10%	20.90%	Wealth Creation
'84	6.4%	4.2%	7.5%	102.0%	5.0%	-21.80%	6.30%	15.43%	7.90%	5.00%	Wealth Creation
'85	2.7%	4.1%	7.2%	120.0%	5.4%	8.72%	31.10%	30.10%	8.70%	53.00%	Wealth Creation
'86	2.5%	1.1%	6.9%	160.0%	5.3%	24.00%	18.00%	24.00%	11.00%	66.80%	Wealth Creation

Source: U.S. Bureau of Labor Statistics, U.S. Bureau of Economics Analysis Survey of Current Business, U.S. Common Stock Index referenced to Standards & Poors 500 Index, E,A,FE Index provided by Morgan Stanley Capital International Perspective.
Assistance with this Chart provided by Jeffrey K. Pashe, Suttons Bay, MI, Colleen M. Curtin, Omena, MI, and Financial & Investment Planning, Ltd., Suttons Bay, MI.

Investment	@ -	_____
Cash Flow From Investment	@	_____
Value of Investment End of Period	@ +	_____
Taxes Paid on Investment Earnings	@ -	_____
Value of Investment After Taxes	@	_____
Less Inflation	@	_____ %
Value of Investment After Inflation and Taxes Total Return	@ +	_____

Fig. 11-1. Simplified method of figuring investment total returns.

performance. If your investments are in a retirement plan, you should expect returns of 4-8 percent after inflation. Figure 11-1 shows a simple method of figuring investment returns.

Table 11-2 shows the importance of favorable compound returns on your investment portfolios. Notice that the difference after 25 years between having a 10 percent return or a 12 percent return makes a difference in your portfolio of over 40 percent, while the difference in compound return is only a difference of 20 percent. Thus, by earning just a few more percent in returns over that period, you end up with thousands more in your pocket.

Table 11-2
The Important of Favorable Compound Return in Your
Investments—$10,000. Annual Contribution

Years to Retirement	5 % Compound Return	10% Compound Return	12% Compound Return	15% Compound Return
05	$ 58,019.	$ 67,156.	$71,152.	$ 77,537.
10	132,068.	175,312.	196,546.	233,493.
15	226,575.	349,497.	417,533.	547,175.
25	501,135.	1,081,818.	1,493,339.	2,447,120.
35	$ 948,383.	$ 2,981,268.	$ 4,834,631.	$ 10,133,457.

Table 11-3
Inflation Effects on Your Investments: The Value of $ 1,000,000.
in Today's Purchasing Power at Various Rates of Inflation

End of year	@ 5%	@ 8%	@ 10%	@ 14%
05	$ 783,530.	$ 680,580.	$ 620,920.	$ 519,370.
10	$ 613,910.	$ 463,190.	$ 385,540.	$ 269,740.
15	$ 481,020.	$ 315,240.	$ 239,390.	$ 140,100.
20	$ 295,300.	$ 146,020.	$ 92.300.	$ 37,790.
25	$ 181,290.	$ 67,630.	$ 35,580.	$ 10,190.

Many individuals become complacent about their investment portfolios. They go year after year with mediocre performance, never exploring any alternatives until it is too late. It is just as important for a portfolio of modest size to have favorable returns as it is for a portfolio of substantial size and value. The time to get serious about your investment portfolio is not after it is substantial, but rather at the beginning stages of setting up your portfolio, whether it is in your IRA, your retirement plan, or personal portfolios.

Table 11-3 shows the inflation effects on an investment fund value of one million dollars, and the total purchasing power lost at various rates of inflation averaging between 5 and 14 percent. Do not get discouraged by these tables since if inflation averages at a high rate of return you are able to keep your practice incomes rising even moderately while being able to save the difference in your retirement plans toward wealth accumulation with proper investments, you will have a good chance of beating inflation.

At the end of the book in the Appendix there are useful tables that you can use to help show you how compound returns can work in your favor. Use these tables in your own financial planning.

Investment Strategies and Investments Forms

12

Once you have earned an income you have two choices: you can spend your money or save it. If you save it you must decide where to invest that money, i.e., in a portfolio of assets designed to serve as a store of value.

Chapters 15 and 16 will deal with Portfolio Management and Portfolio Constructions. This chapter will deal with the specific investments that you may place in your portfolios.

In Chapter 11 you learned that the economy is cyclical, and you should combine the information you learned in Chapter 10 with the information in this chapter to start developing your own philosophy so that you can construct a portfolio to achieve your specific investment goals.

Chapter 13 will deal specifically with risks as will this chapter somewhat; however, you must clear your mind of all investment concepts and realize that all investments have risks. Your job is to manage that risk.

We will discuss specific investment forms that you should look at as tools for you to use in your portfolio to achieve your specific investment goals and objectives. This chapter deals with security analysis where by you consider each individual asset by itself while in Chapters 15 and 16 you will deal with Portfolio Management, which takes the aggregate view.

These investments will range from those investments that have predictable returns such as savings accounts, money market investments, CDs, short-term bonds, annuities, treasury notes, etc., to those investments that have extremely unpredictable returns. Investments that have predictable returns have a great degree of liquidity, i.e., you can sell them quickly without taking any loss.

Most popular forms of predictable return investments are savings accounts, money market accounts, CDs, short-term government bonds and cash. These investments also act very well as a safe harbor during periods when you should not be in the longer term oriented investments or those investments that have more unpredictable returns. These investments should be utilized when you cannot figure out what type of investment cycle we are currently in or in periods when you are not sure to invest.

You learned in Chapter 11 your investment goals should be favorable total return. If you figure out the total return after taxes and inflation on these predictable investments you will find that returns are often negative or at best modest. However, don't let that bother you if your portfolio sits in those type of investments for awhile, as other assets that are more long term oriented may be losing substantial values because of principal loss.

Tables 12-1 and 12-2 illustrate each investment and make comments regarding them.

Table 12-1
Safe Harbor Investments: Mature in Less than 1 Year and are Very Liquid

Investment	Investment Characteristics	Liquidity	Notes
Bank money market funds or money market mutual funds. Note, a mutual fund is a method of owning money market securities.	Pool of assets investing for capital preservation, total liquidity and yields.	Complete—most offer checkwriting and wire redemption.	Excellent parking place for capital. Stick to high-grade funds or government funds during crisis or wealth destruction economy.
T-bills.	Short term bonds issues by U.S. Government. Mature in less than 1 year.	Excellent.	Don't buy 1 year maturities if interest rates are rising, but short term notes, i.e., 1 month to 3 months. Always see if money market funds are a better deal.
Short term C.D.'s negotiable and nonnegotiable.	Short term debt instruments issued by banks and savings and loans. Negotiables can be sold prior to maturity without early withdrawal penalty. Nonnegotiables may have penalties.	Excellent for negotiables. Okay for non-negotiables.	Check out the C.D.'s fees for early withdrawal. Only buy if they have U.S. Government, F.S.L.I.C. or F.D.I.C. insurance.
Short term corporate bonds or paper.	Short term debt instruments of corporations maturing in less than 1 year.	Excellent for large amounts.	Usually better to go with a money market fund that owns this type of investment.

Note: Safe harbor investments are to be used when the market for long term oriented assets such as common stocks, long term bonds, real estate, metals, etc., seems unfavorable.

Table 12-2
The Universe of Equity (Ownership) Investments

Investment	Investment Characteristics	Liquidity	Ability to Sell Quickly; Marketability	Primary Rewards	Primary Risks	Notes
Real estate, "housing"	Purchase of single family or multiple family housing as an investment	Low	Low	Income, price appreciation, ability to leverage, tax benefits	Vacancies, can be hard to sell, leverage can cause problems, property can lose value and will depreciate, competition	Well selected, prudently purchased properties can be a fine investment. Look at each "deal" individually
Real estate, commercial	Purchase of commercial buildings to lease or rent to companies	Low	Low	Income, price appreciation, ability to leverage, tax benefits	Same as above, may be very hard to release or re-rent, tenant could go bankrupt, competition	Same as above. Check out your tenant
Real estate, raw land	Purchase of raw land	Low to terrible	Low to terrible	Price appreciation	High carrying costs, i.e., taxes, interest if leveraged, no tax advantages, no income, can be hard to sell or impossible, zoning problems, etc.	This is a high risk investment. Investigate why this will be good investment before you buy
Real estate, farms	Purchase of real estate for agricultural development and utilization	Low	Low	Income, price appreciation	High labor costs, high costs of doing business, cyclical business	

Investment	Description		Income	Rewards	Risks	Comments
Oil and gas, coal (energy)	Purchase of oil and gas, coal reserves or development or exploration of reserves	Low	Depends upon amount of oil and gas you own and type of ownership	Rewards could be income, price appreciation, can be inflation hedge, tax benefits	If drilling, deal could be dry hole (s). Price could go down; you could lose all of your investment	Each deal must be looked at individually. All deals are risky; however, in some, you could lose all of your investment
Gold, silver, precious metals	Ownership of gold, silver, precious metals; through outright ownership or common stocks of companies mining or processing metals	Low	Low to excellent	Inflation hedge, price appreciation	Price could go down, if leveraged you could lose your entire investment monies	There are many ways to own this type of investment, some are very speculative; usually best to stick to common stocks, or outright *delivered* ownership
Collectibles, coins, stamps	Buying collectibles for price appreciation	Low	Low to poor	Price appreciation, inflation hedge	High markup, manias, substantial price declines are possible, counterfeits	Many collectibles such as coins may be due for a substantial price decline because of stong manias in the marketplace and ability to manipulate prices
Diamonds, gems	Diamonds, gems	Low	Low to terrible	Price appreciation, inflation hedge	High markup, manias, substantial price declines are possible, counterfeits	Diamonds and gems have been known to go down or up faster than blood pressure; require patience

(Table 12-2 Continues.)

(*Table 12-2 Continued.*)

Investment	Investment Characteristics	Liquidity	Ability to Sell Quickly; Marketability	Primary Rewards	Primary Risks	Notes
Small, emerging growth common stocks	Stocks in companies that are small and immature. It is easier for a company to go from $10,000,000. in sales to $100,000,000. than it is for a company to go from $100,000,000 to $1,000,000,000.	Low	Moderate to good	Price appreciation and growth to a seasoned company	Business market, company could go bankrupt, shares could become over-valued	Well-selected growth common stocks have been excellent long-term investments for the patient investor
Common stocks in seasoned companies	Stocks representing ownership of larger or more mature companies	Usually OK; however, there will be price volatility	Good to excellent	Price appreciation, dividend growth, current dividends (total returns)	Company could go bankrupt or come on bad times	Common stocks in seasoned mature companies have performed very well in many economies
Warrants	Carry the right to own a stock at a set price; within a specific period	Low	Moderate to good	Low cost, price appreciation	Same as common stocks; however, you don't own stock, you own only the right to buy the stock at a set price. Time period may run out	
Calls	Carry the right to buy a stock at a pre-determined price within a period of time; usually less than 6 months	Low	Moderate to poor	Low Cost	Time might run out before stock goes up. Same as common stock	Selling covered calls can be a profitable way to increase returns

13

Investment Strategies and Investment Risks

I looked at a client as he dumped a little bag of diamonds on to the table. The diamonds scattered, and I asked the client, "How much did you pay for these?" He said, "$23,000." I asked, "Why did you buy them?" He answered, "I bought them because diamonds up until 1981 had gone up about six times in value over the prior few short years, and I thought I could make a lot of money by investing in them." I asked, "Would you invest in them now?" And he said, "No, who would want to invest in anything that went from $23,000 down to $3,000?" I asked, "Why would anyone want to invest in something that went from $3,000 up to $23,000?" He answered, "Because they had good growth."

Most people who have invested money have horror stories similar to the one told by this client. We have a tendency to always want to go with the winning investment that has a spectacular performance over a period. It is our human nature to want to go with a "winner" and the investment sellers will spend most of their time explaining the rewards of the investment they want to sell you based on its track record. If an investment you are considering has gone straight up, look out, back away, and examine that investment carefully before you invest.

Risk is the uncertainty that the anticipated return will be achieved. Note that a key word in this phrase is "anticipated returns." When you make an investment you should anticipate the returns that you expect. Do you expect that the total return of that investment over the next 5 years will be 14 percent—that the investment will double over the next 6 years? Do you expect that the investment will give you a 10 percent cash flow each year, plus a 2 or 3 percent price appreciation? Once you have determined what your anticipated returns will be, you must analyze the specific investment risks that will affect the potential rewards. For example, had the client purchased the diamonds, correctly, he would have analyzed what forces would continue to make diamonds rise spectacularly, i.e., commercial use, use as jewelry, etc. If he had analyzed the diamond market, he would have realized that the diamond market is very easily manipulated, and very price sensitive, and that there were diamond companies spring-ing up left and right throughout the country by people who had little or no experience in that marketplace. If there had been proper analyzation of the risk revolving around the potential rewards of a diamond investment that investor probably would not have made that investment or would have said, "I'm only going to risk a few thousand dollars of my portfolio in this investment, rather than taking a substantial piece of the action."

There are four basic types of risks. They are business risks, financial risks, market risks, and purchasing power risks.

Business risk is associated with the risk inherent in whatever the busi-ness involves itself in specifically. Naturally, each business does not have equal risk. For example, with an investment in a fledgling new computer company, you will have to compete with the likes of IBM and Apple, and would have substantially more risk than an investment in an electric utility.

When you are analyzing an investment representing an ownership in-terest in a business either through partnership or common stock, you must analyze the specific risks of that business by reviewing its competition, specific products, markets, etc.

The second primary risk is financial risk. Financial risk comes from the fact that all assets must be financed, either through creditors (debt), owners (shareholders), or a combination of both. Naturally, borrowing funds creates a greater element of risk because creditors must be paid in-terest and principal in a timely matter. A creditor can also demand other terms, such as collateral, or restrictions on dividends that increase the risks of any business debt.

Business and financial risks are often called unsystematic risks, which means that the risk inherent in these types of enterprises are specific to the individual firms, individual company or endeavor, rather than the risks inherent in the market as a whole. Unsystematic risk can be significantly reduced through the utilization of *diversification*.

Two other risk types must be understood and considered. Systematic risk means that the market values of assets tend to rise and fall together, and there is a systematic relationship between the prices of an individual security and the market overall. For that reason, market risk is called sys-tematic risk. An example of this would be if you purchased an investment in an extremely favorable company that had an excellent balance sheet, good marketing ideas, and an extremely saleable product, only to watch the price of that security fall with the rest of the stock market, although maybe not as much. Market risk is not just inherent in the common stock market, you will see it in real estate, coins, horses, stamps, precious met-als, gem stones, etc. While you can reduce the impact of financial risk by diversification, market risk cannot be avoided.

The fourth area of risk is purchasing power risk. Purchasing power risk is that risk associated with inflation. Inflation is the loss of purchasing power due to rising prices. If the prices of goods and services rise, purchasing power of your assets and the income generated with it is reduced. Purchasing power risk is the risk that inflation will ruin the buying power of your assets and income.

To protect yourself from purchasing power risk, utilizing investments that have an anticipated return higher than inflation can prove to offset these risks. Thus, if inflation is anticipated to be 8 percent and you can earn 10-12 percent on your money, you are naturally beating inflation at least before taxes. The problem is, however, that higher yields usually mean bearing more risk.

Thus, we come to the main point of this chapter—as an investor your primary duty is to manage risk. You cannot avoid risk. By doing nothing, holding cash, or putting your money in savings accounts and treasury bills, you are still bearing some element of risk, i.e., purchasing power risk. When you evaluate your investments, you must analyze each of the specific risks and its inherent effect on that specific investment, be it business, financial, market, and/or purchasing power risk.

Regarding systematic risk, economic, political, and sociological changes all affect systematic risk. Systematic risk is found to varying degrees in almost all securities, because as mentioned earlier, comparable securities move together in a systematic manner.

It is the opinion of the author, however, that in analyzing risks, you must primarily seek to avoid purchasing assets whose price has appreciated substantially due to a mania. John Maynard Keynes in his book, *The General Theory of Employment, Interest and Money* (New York, Harcourt Brace Jovanovich. 1936.), argued that short-run speculation, not long-run expectations is the key determinant of stock prices. This is a quote from Keynes about money managers.

> Most of these persons are in fact largely concerned not with making superior long-term forecasts of the probable yield of an investment over its whole life, but with forseeing changes in the conventional basis of valuation a short time ahead of the general public. They are concerned not with what the investment is really worth to a man who buys it (for keeps), but with what the market will value it at under the influence of mass psychology three months or a year hence. Thus, the professional investor is forced to concern himself with the anticipation of impending changes in the news or in the atmosphere of the kind by which experience shows the "mass psychology" of the market is most influenced. (pp. 154-155, with permission.)

London, in the early part of 1524, was a city in panic. The soothsayers had said that on February 1 the Thymes would suddenly rise from its banks to such an extent as to destroy most all of London by engulfing the city and sweeping away thousands of homes. This horror was described in great detail by the gypsies, star gazers, numerologists, and soon even the most respected and level-headed of the population began to believe the soothsayers convincing speculation that London would soon be swept away. St. Bartholomew built a huge tower high on a hill, put enough provisions and supplies for 2 months, and hired 700 boats manned by expert rowers just in case it rose above his tower. As February 1 drew near, nobles and clergy followed the thousands of people who departed London awaiting that fateful date.

When the ill-fated date arrived, a few braver souls stayed behind to watch, because the soothsayers had predicted that the river would rise slowly and thus they could escape before they were swept away. When the fateful hour came, much to the consternation of those watching, nothing happened, the tide ebbed and flowed as it had always done, and quickly an awareness spread over all the good people that they had been had. To be safe, however, many stayed the night and continued to watch. The next morning the river continued to flow peacefully along its banks and the crowd was boiling with fury. Many threatened to throw the pack of soothsayers in the river. Fortunately, the prophets were prepared, and by a clever maneuver, not unlike our modern day economists, the previous night these technicians had found a minute error. It was a minor oversight, naturally. The great flood would occur not in 1524, but in 1624. Thus, the townspeople could go home, although only for another hundred years.

Acts such as this have been played throughout history. This mania properly describes the manias that happen in the investment markets. Manias do not just happen in the common stock market, you will see it in many small towns in the real estate markets. You will see it in land speculations that have happened in Florida and California and these manias not only affect the ignorant, but also affect the highly educated and intelligent individual.

Table 13-1 shows some of the favorite investments from different eras, so that you can see the substantial price of manias that have happened, from the tulip bulb mania in 1637 to the manias that have affected common stocks in the 1960s and 70s.

Chapter 15 will deal with portfolio management and how to structure your portfolio and manage the specific risks of investments.

It is extremely important that you understand that the bottom line of this chapter is that all investments have risks. It is your job when you make an investment to manage and analyze risk, and if that risk is properly managed, you have the potential to create substantial rewards for yourself.

Table 13-1
Market Favorites From Different Eras

	High Price	Low Price	Price Decline from High (percent)
Holland, 1637			
Semper Augustis (tulip bulbs)	5,500*	50*	99
England, 1720			
South Sea Company	1,050†	129†	88
France, 1720			
Mississippi Company	18,000‡	200‡	99
USA 1929-1932			
Burroughs	97	6¼	86
General Motors	115	7⅝	94
Montgomery Ward	158	3½	98
USA 1961-1962			
AMF	66⅜	10	84
Brunswick	4⅞	13⅛	82
Texas Instruments	207	49	76
USA 1971-1972			
Avon	140	18⅝	87
Disney	119⅛	16⅝	86
Levitz Furniture	40¼	3⅞	90
Litton Industries	104	15	86
National Student Marketing	143	3½	98
Polaroid	149½	14⅛	91

* Florins
† Pounds sterling
‡ Livres
From Fabozzi, Frank J: *Readings in Investment Management*. Richard D. Irwin, Inc., Homewood, IL. With permission.

14

Investment Strategies—Uncle Sam Wants You to Succeed (Tax Planning)

The Congress shall have the power to lay and collect tax on incomes from whatever source arrived without apportionment among the several states and without regard to any census or enumeration.

The 16th Amendment to the Constitution, 1913

Many people will do almost anything to avoid paying taxes, even risking their own financial health. This chapter will deal with tax favored investments and the utilization of tax favored investments to help you in your overall investment planning.

It must be understood that the first tax planning strategies that you should consider were those outlined in Chapter 8. The uses of business forms and tax-favored trusts are virtually riskless financial transactions when compared to using investments to help reduce taxes and create wealth. After you properly utilize business forms, retirement plan trusts, and other types of trusts the utilization of tax-favored investments must be considered.

Prior to 1987, tax-sheltered investments offered significant tax savings to most high income individuals. Now, however, the use of passive tax-shelter losses to shelter anything other than passive income is severely restricted. Also with a new top tax rate of 28 percent, the losses you may get are not as juicy as pre-1987's 50 percent top tax rate.

While prior to 1987 a significant part of the economics of tax-favored investment was tax related, now more than ever you must look at the economics of each investment.

Tax-favored investments are not supposed to be poor investments that lose money and thus taxes. *Tax-favored investments should be extremely profitable investments that will make you substantial economic gains in addition to giving you tax benefits.* How do you tell the glitter from the gold in tax-

tax-favored investments? Table 14-1 lists some questions that you need to ask regarding any tax-favored investments that you are considering for your own personal investment portfolio. In addition, you should seek competent financial planning help and tax advice regarding any tax shelter investment. You must discuss your financial goals and plans in depth with a tax attorney, accountant, or another financial advisor familiar with such investments before you make any specific investments in tax shelters.

Conceptually, when you invest in a tax shelter you are investing in a business. That business may be real estate, oil and gas, cable television, or leasing airplanes. Your first decision must be: Would you invest in that business as a business if there were no tax advantages involved? You must decide whether the business is viable without the tax advantages.

Once you decide your new endeavor should be profitable, you should analyze it in a wholistic manner—looking at all the advantages, investment risks, and rewards. After you are convinced the project will make money, then look at its structure to see whether you will be able to share in the profits equitably. We will assume that you are smart enough and lucky enough to buy into a business that will be profitable. However, you must pay very careful attention to what you will get out of the deal and whether you will properly participate in the deal commensurate with the risks. Thus, you not only have to invest in a favorable investment deal, you have to make sure that the deal is also fair to you.

If you buy a partnership, you should check out the general partners, fees, and partnership expenses, and how profits are divided up. Naturally, answers to these questions will vary from one partnership to another. There are generally five people involved in each different tax-sheltered investment. First, the investor; second, the investment manufacturer; third, the business manager; fourth, the salesperson; and fifth, the advisor to the investor.

The Investor

Each limited partnership will be designed specifically for an individual investor with specific investment needs. In the offering memorandum given out by the investment manufacturer it will outline who that specific investment is designed for. You should fit the description of the ideal candidate for that investment as outlined in their prospectus/offering material.

If you are in a limited partnership, you will be entirely passive and, generally, once you buy into a partnership it is very costly and expensive to get out of the deal. Make sure it fits your goals well.

The Manufacturer

The manufacturer, (often called the promoter), is the company or people who put the investment deal together. The manufacturer is the

Table 14-1
Questions You Should Ask About the Tax-favored Investments

1. What will this partnership own?

2. How much will the properties the partnership is buying cost and is there a fair price?

3. Where will the economic benefits come from? (i.e., tax benefits, appreciation, income, etc.)

4. What assumptions are made about the economic benefits (i.e., tax savings, appreciation and income) and are they reasonable? Why?

5. Is this partnership structured so that I will participate in the (1) expected tax benefits; (2) appreciation; and (3) income, etc.?

6. Does this investment have the "potential" to throw off phantom income? How much? Why?

7. If this is a "blind pool" partnership:
   a. Who will be making the investment decisions?
   b. What is their background?
   c. What is their track record?

8. a. Who will manage the partnership?
   b. What is their background?
   c. What is their track record?
   d. Are they financially strong?

9. a. What is my total limit of liability on this investment?
   b. Is their any chance I will need to add more cash to this deal, and if so, how much?

10. What is the expected life on this investment?

11. If this investment "blows up" and is a disaster, does the general partner/manager have the staying power to properly manage the program to the best advantage of the limited partners, or will the general partner/manager walk away?

12. a. After fees, commissions, mark-ups, interest, and other front-end expenses, how much of my $1 is going to be invested, first, as a percent of equity raised and second, as a percent of the total deal (including debt)?
    b. How will I participate in the profits, cash flow, and appreciation on this program after it is up and running (i.e., how much will I get and how much will the general partner get)?

13. a. Is the general partner taking on substantial risks for its contributuion to the partnership?
    b. Will the general partner have a strong incentive to make the program work both economically and to maintain a good reputation?
    c. What specific economic incentive does the general partner have to make this deal work?

14. a. Do I fit to a T the offering memorandums explanation of Who should invest?
    b. Does my advisor agree?

15. Why is this investment better for me than another oil and gas deal, a growth mutual fund, a variable annuity, another leasing deal, or another real estate deal, etc.?

16. If this is a multiple write-off deal ($2 for $1 invested), do I have a letter from a major CPA or law firm stating that they feel that the tax benefits will flow to me as advised?

17. Do I have a letter from my tax shelter salesperson answering each of these questions?

18. Am I properly diversifying my tax sheltered investment portfolio or am I risking it all on one investment?

19. Are my IRA's fully funded, have I taken full advantage of TSA's, TSCA's, Pension and Profit Sharing Plan, business form, etc., to save taxes?

20. Does this investment fit into my overall financial plan?

21. Has my tax shelter salesman and financial planner gone over this questionnaire with me?

entrepreneur. When you read an offering memorandum or prospectus, you will not find someone named the manufacturer or promoter. The promoter or manufacturer is often the general partner of the deal and takes on many of the risks that are involved in the deal.

The general partner is generally well compensated for the risks and the time that it takes to put a deal together. Many types of tax-sheltered deals have substantial expenses before you even hear about the specific investment. For example, in real estate the manufacturer will search out projects, develop plans, obtain financing, and perhaps form a syndicate to help sell the project. In many cases he or she may already own the investment before you even hear about it. The general partner will run the business, so it is very important that the general partner know his or her stuff and is competent. There are some corporate general partners that have experts who specialize in each specific type of business or enterprise in which you may be investing. The professionals who take on the risks and run the business have unlimited liability when it comes to the partnerships, debts, liability, etc.

The manufacturer will usually receive front-end fees, management fees, and residual fees. The front-end fees are those charged to get the business set up. They may be reimbursements for out-of-pocket expenses such as accounting, marketing expenses (commissions), printing and legal expenses. The manufacturer and promoter may also get part of the profits, including management fees charged for the ongoing management of the business or enterprise. Sometimes management fees are fixed expenses or they may be a percentage of profits or gross income. These fees are carefully structured into the deal since it is important that they are deductible to the limited partners.

The last is the residual fee. These are taken at the end of the deal when the project is sold. For example, a general partner might take 10 percent off the top of sale proceeds in a property, plus a percentage of the balance over a minimum return to the investors, or he or she may have just a fixed residual fee. With tax-favored investments, each deal will have a different compensation structure and different fees and expenses. The prospectus and offering memorandum will explain fees in detail.

Business Manager

The third player is the manager, or operator, of the business, who could also be the general partner, promoter, and/or investment manufacturer. If the promoter or the manufacturer does not have the expertise, he or she may hire an expert, as discussed earlier, who manages the business or he or she may contract out for specific services.

Salesperson

The fourth player is the salesperson. There are many tax shelter salespeople. There are insurance agents who turned instant financial planners, brokerage house people who found the commissions involved in tax shelters were substantially greater at 5-10 percent than those paid on stock and bond trades. There are also financial planners who carefully analyze your situation and make recommendations in writing based on your needs. These planners may or may not be independent of brokerage houses. Often they work for themselves or a small broker/dealership and/or financial planning firm. Whoever recommends a deal to you should be familiar with tax-favored investments and advise you specifically on the tax-favored investments that will help you obtain your financial goals. This is not to say that insurance salespeople, stockbrokers, or a person working for the specific promoter cannot provide you with good advice. Because commissions are very favorable in tax shelter deals, it is extremely important that you understand who is on your side.

When working with a salesperson, discover if he or she has more than one shelter deal that he or she can put you into and ask for an explanation of why that specific investment is better for your situation than another. For example, if the salesperson recommends real estate, ask why an operating leasing investment, cable television, oil and gas, or another specific investment would not be better for your situation.

The Advisor to the Investor

The fifth person is the advisor to you as an investor. A fee that you pay to your tax advisor, tax attorney, accountant or an independent financial planning firm or a financial planner who is familiar with tax-favored investments is the best investment you can make *before* you invest your money in a specific deal. The fees you pay to a good advisor may be tax deductible, and in most cases, will make sure you do not get into a litany of problems. You should not look to a tax advisor to help you with a decision about the business and how that business should be run. A tax advisor should be able to give you objective advice about whether that investment can specifically help you in your situation. Thus, if you decided that you would like to get involved in a tax-sheltered investment, a good advisor can help you decide if an investment's tax benefits are good, and which one is best for you.

Secondly, a tax shelter advisor can look at the assumptions made by the promoter to see if they are in line or not. This information should be in the offering memorandum and/or prospectus. If it is not in either of those, then you should get some specific information from the investment company, even if it is a blind pool or investment that does not own any specific property yet. You and your advisor must decide whether the goals and objectives of the tax-sheltered investment will have a good chance of being realized and if you will have a good chance of realizing the benefits of that particular deal. Look out for blind pools especially in oil and gas programs. There is saying, "Blind pools are for the blind fools."

Having worked personally with clients who invest in tax favored investments, both on the selling side and just advising clients, it is important to understand when you are dealing with a tax attorney or accountant that your advisors stick to their expertise. For example, what is a reasonable fee to the promoter or salesperson may seem too large to your independent advisor. I have seen investors turn down a deal because they felt the fees and commissions were a little bit too high, even though they were a small percentage of total partnership capital raised, or even though the tax favored investment appeared to have extremely favorable economic and tax benefits.

After careful analysis, if your advisors feel the deal is good overall, with sound economic potential, the final decision is still yours.

In addition to tax analysis, analyzing the economic merits of the deal is a whole new problem. Usually investment advisors who specialize in tax shelters can help you analyze both the tax considerations and the economic considerations. Often someone that is trained in economics or investment analysis can help you look at that investment like a business and help you ascertain the risk and potential rewards of making that investment. You will pay for investment advice such as this; however, you will receive much more than what you pay them. Look out if your salesperson tells you whom to call for expertise. Salespeople want your business, and some will pay grandly to get it. Frequently, in the course of selling tax shelters, kickbacks are paid. Accountants and lawyers often will bring investors together with a promoter or salesperson. Without the client knowing it, the salesperson may give part of his commission to the advisor in return for the introduction. The split sometimes can be fifty-fifty. This practice is unethical and illegal, but it is often done. Often these payments are called referral or representative payments or fees by the salesperson.

Many accounting firms have policies against fees, commissions, or kickbacks, etc. of this type, however, the fee may be paid specifically to the individual accountant or lawyer in the form other than a cash payment such as a trip to Hawaii, a new color TV, a sailboat, etc. If your tax-sheltered salesperson advises you to go to a specific attorney or accountant, it is very important you ask the salesperson (whether he or she is called a financial planner, salesperson, broker, or advisor) if they will be paid any money, because you invest in the deal.

If they will receive compensation if you invest in the deal, then you should go to another accountant or attorney, or at best, use trusted advisors that are familiar with your specific situation. Your advisor may not be a tax-sheltered expert; however, if he or she has been able to give good advice in the past, a practical no-nonsense person who is interested in your well-being is much better than an expert who is going to receive a substantial fee if you invest in the deal.

Once you invest in the tax shelter, your money will go to pay expenses and to purchase specific assets. Most expenses and most of the equity raised in a deal will come from you as a limited partner. In fact, there is a joke about this, although dry, that goes something like this: In the beginning the limited partners have all the money, the general partners have none, and at the end of the deal the general partners have all the money, and the limited partners have none.

Just as there are medical "quacks," or so-called health care "professionals" on the fringes of medical competence and ethics who hurt the legitimate physicians and health care professionals, so there are equivalents in the tax-favored investment area. I can personally visualize many executives at my own broker/dealer who manufactured many quality tax-favored investments that have been extremely successful and made great investments for their clients, rolling their eyes and being upset by my last joke since they take pride in putting together professional, honest deals with excellent economics. These professionals can be found in many organizations and when investing in deals, it is a good idea to invest in an organization that has a reputation to defend.

HOW A TAX SHELTER SHELTERS TAXES

Tax-favored investments, as we discussed, are generally businesses, except for annuities, municipal bonds, etc. Businesses are allowed to deduct all expenses that have to do with running that business. Thus, the basic business equation of business—business income minus deductions equals profit or loss—is the basic equation that a tax-sheltered promoter will manipulate in order to provide specific investment benefits to its subscribers. Since a tax-sheltered investment gives you losses in the years when deductions exceed income, often these losses will be structured in such a way as to maximize tax advantages to you as an investor. Often these tax deductions are received early in the deal with (sometimes taxable) profits being realized later, often after the deal is sold.

However, beware of those passive partnership tax shelter losses because generally after 1986 they only will shelter other passive partnership income and not your earned income.Thus, you could end up with a lot of deductions with nothing to deduct them against, since most physicians' incomes comes from their professional skills and not investments.

This tax law game changes almost annually, and some of the deals as stated may throw-off tax sheltered losses that may not be able to be used to shelter certain types of income. This is why it is extremely important that you always meet with your accountant to make sure that you will be able to realize the tax benefits of investing in any specific tax-favored plan. You must explore the alternative minimum tax (AMT) whether or not there is going to be excess investor interest, etc., and only a trained professional can help.

If you are in a 30 percent tax bracket and your tax sheltered losses are $10,000 you may save $3,000 in taxes, depending on whether you get to use the losses. As you can see by this example, there are tax incentives to invest in tax-favored investments; however, just because a loss may be realized on your tax investment you may not get to use it because of the tax laws and your specific situation.

Another form of deduction you may get is in the form of a credit. A credit is better than a deduction because in a credit each dollar of credit offsets, dollar for dollar, your tax. Thus, if you have to pay $10,000 in taxes and you have a $10,000 tax credit, the $10,000 tax credit would completely wipe out the $10,000 tax liability.

All stories have good news and bad news and since personal income minus tax-sheltered loss equals income subject to tax, a tax-sheltered deal could increase your tax liability when the investment starts making money. Remember, you invested in the deal to make money, and once your deal starts making money you may want to sell it, gift it, or use another strategy so that you do not have to pay the taxes on those profits.

It is extremely expensive to get out of a tax-shelter partnership and you may have to take a substantial loss if you sell before it reaches term, i.e., they sell the building or the last drop of partnership oil is sold. Often these tax-favored investments that are throwing off substantial taxable income can be sold to a pension or profit sharing plan, gifted to an individual who is in a low tax bracket and thus, instead of having the taxable benefits taxed at your high tax bracket, they may be taxed at a zero percent tax bracket as in the case of an IRA, Keogh, or pension plan, or in a low tax bracket of your child over age 14, your parents, etc.

Some tax-favored deals can throw off phantom income. Phantom income is income that is realized from a deal that has no cash flow to you to help pay the taxes. In Table 14-1 there are some questions that we suggest you ask the promoter. For example, "Is there potential for phantom income?" Phantom income can be very devastating since you could end up with a substantial taxable income generated from an investment with no cash received to pay the taxes on that profit from the venture.

Whenever you go into a highly leveraged tax-favored investment there is a chance of phantom income. Although it can happen in nonleveraged deals the risk of phantom income is very substantial in highly leveraged deals.

Some deals are structured so that they will throw off phantom income in the future. If phantom income is anticipated, however, you must plan for it and the deal can still work out as a favorable investment.

Judge Learned Hand, the famous New York State jurist, said, "Anyone may so arrange his affairs that his taxes shall be as low as possible. He is not bound to choose that pattern which best pays the treasury."

Senator Bryan P. Harrison, of Mississippi, a former chairman of the Senate Finance Committee said it this way, "There is nothing that says a man has to take a toll bridge across the river when there is a free bridge nearby."

The continued growth of tax-sheltered investments is a rational response by some taxpayers and an irrational response by others. A tax-favored investment is a rational response to high taxes if it is carefully selected and if, after taxes, it can provide returns greater than those that could have been expected from an alternative investment.

In tax-favored investments generally you cannot do much more than defer your ultimate tax liability to some day in the future and often you will hear "pay me now, or pay me later." There is, however, substantial incentive to pay later than now, since if you paid later you could benefit from price appreciation, inflation, and on the use of the current tax savings.

Table 14-2 illustrates some of the most common tax-favored investments. In using this table, first you must decide what your specific investment goals are and what you want that investment to provide you with. For example, do you want tax-favored income? Do you want high tax write-offs that can help shelter income from other partnership investments? Do you want low risks? Do you want investments that have predictable returns? Are you a high risk individual who wants to take some flyers and have the tax laws reduce your initial investment by tax savings in that deal? Table 14-2 will help you decide what specific investment is best for you and make it easier for you to do planning with your advisors.

In summary, tax-favored investments can be great investments if; the specific investments that you buy fit your needs; if the deal is structured so that you can realize the substantial economic benefits that could be realized by the deal; if the investment ends up making substantial profits; if you receive and participate in those tax losses and profits as you originally thought you would; and, if you hold that investment long enough to realize the economic gains of the investment. Most tax-favored investments are long term oriented and, thus you should be willing to hold on to that investment for substantially longer than the average person holds on to the average spouse.

Table 14-2
Most Common Tax-Favored Investments

Investment	Description of Investment	Goal of Investment	Type of Investor	Potential for Growth	Primary Risk	Primary Reward	Notes
Annuities (variable)	Income, dividends, and growth all grow tax deferred. Has tremendous investment flexibility. Usually companies have stock, bond, government bond, and money market account to choose from.	Tax-deferred accumulation of wealth. Investment goal depends upon type your annuity invests in.	Investor who has a time horizon of 5 years or so and wants to accumulate wealth in a tax wise manner. The investor can be from conservative to aggressive since variable annuities offer accounts that invest from stocks to money market funds.	Depends upon account you choose (i.e., excellent for stock accounts, none for money market accounts).	Risk associated with investment in your variable annuity.	Rewards will depend upon how well you choose your variable annuities investments. Some variable annuities have had excellent results.	See above notes for fixed annuities and variable annuities that allow switching between the family of variable annuity investments have been very popular. For example, you can switch from stocks, to bonds, etc. as the economy changes.
Oil and gas drilling	Partnership drills to find oil and gas reserves.	Some tax advantages. Hopefully, partners will have a gusher.	Aggressive investors who don't want to fly to Las Vegas.	Excellent	Loss of all money invested in the program. Dry holes.		Remember, if it is a good prospect, you *never* hear about it; if it is an OK prospect, you *may* hear about it; if it is a poor prospect, you *will* hear about it (oilmen keep the good prospects for themselves).

Cattle breeding	Purchase of cows in hopes that they increase in value, multiply, etc.	Tax deductions over period of years, economic returns from sale of cattle.	Farmers or investors who believe that the risk/reward ratio is favorable for their investment situation.	Yes	Cyclical market price of cattle, costs of feed and maintenance of cattle, floods, drought, sickness, and so on, could wipe out your herd.	Tax benefits, flexibility in taking back gain (hopefully) from sale of herd.	Check the program and check out management. Don't get rustled; assure yourself you actually paid a fair price for cows and management.
Research and development, technology, medical science partnerships, movies, art reproductions, cable TV, and so on.	Varies; each partnership is different.	Varies with partnerships.		Varies with partnership.	Management risk, tax risk, economic risk, business cycle risk, will vary with partnerships.	Tax benefits, cash flow, capital gains will vary with partnerships.	Look out for "private deals" not offered through large broker-dealer. If offered by a "financial planner," check him or her out thoroughly.
Oil and gas-income programs	Partnership buys proven oil and gas reserves at a discount to provide favorable returns.	High cash flow that could increase or decrease depending upon the price of oil and gas.	Investor wishing to have investment returns tied directly to price of oil and gas. Provides good cash flow.	Excellent	Management risks. Declining oil and gas prices could interrupt or decrease cash flow. Leveraged programs are hurt substantially by lower oil and gas prices.	High tax-favored cash flow, inflation hedge.	For diversification in a retirement portfolio, oil and gas income partnerships offer some protection from inflation.

(Table 14-2 continues.)

(Table 14-2 continued.)

Investment	Description of Investment	Goal of Investment	Type of Investor	Potential for Growth	Primary Risk	Primary Reward	Notes
Real estate—rental "housing," apartments, condominiums, homes	Purchase of housing to rent out as a business	Tax deferral, tax write-offs. Growth of property values for capital gains income from rents (depends on deal). If program throws off more losses than income, make sure you will be able to use losses.	Depends on "deal." Each deal or partnership has different goals. Structure of investment and type of specific property will impact your returns and benefits.	Moderate to excellent.	Business risk of not having tenants, rising costs, and so on. No guarantee property will appreciate or be marketable when you choose to sell. Look out for phantom income.	Tax benefits, possible inflation hedge, potential for growth, income.	Each "investment" should be individually analyzed.
Real estate—commercial	Leasing commercial manufacturing or office buildings to receive economic and tax benefits. (Also, hotels and motels puchased for above.)	Tax benefits such as high multiple write-offs in early years, tax-sheltered cash flow, and so on. Also, potential for property to appreciate.	Each specific partnership investment property should be individually analyzed to ascertain risks and potential rewards. For the conservative investor low or no leverage deals can provide excellent income.	Very moderate to excellent.	High economic and tax risks for highly leveraged deals or deals without good tenants. Lease terms should be favorable. Look out for phantom income. Make sure you will benefit if deal has significant tax incentives.	Tax benefits, possible inflation hedge, growth potential. If in limited partnership, add ability to pool capital, possible diversification and limited liability. Income programs can provide excellent tax sheltered cash flow.	Check over the sponsor, the "business," the tenant. Many non-leveraged programs offer excellent cash flow for conservative investors.

Investment	Description	Features	Rating	Risks	Tax/Income Benefits	Comments
Equipment leasing	You as an investor, individually or as a partner, purchase capital assests such as planes, computers, ships, industrial machines, and so on, to be leased to the user of the equipment.	Lessor receives tax benefits and cash flow from lessee. Programs are set up to provide growth, income, or combination of both.	Some programs are structured for the conservative investor. Some programs are highly leveraged to enhance tax benefits to high tax bracket investors. High Leverage = High Risk.	Poor to OK	Lessee may not make payments, leased assets may lose their value. Interest rates may fluctuate. Look out for phantom income.	Tax shelter through investment tax credit, depreciation, business expenses, and so on. Cash flow from lease payments. See your tax advisor before buying a leasing deal.	Some leasing partnerships offer excellent predictable tax benefits and are structured to minimize credit risks. Check out your manager if you are in a partnership.
Municipal bonds, "tax-free bonds," municipal bond trust, and so on	Income from bonds is not taxed by federal government, often not by state or local governments. Issued by municipal governments. After 1986, some bonds that are called Munis' may not be tax free. Check them over and be aware.	Tax-free income.	Investor needing tax-free income. Conservative investor may use tax-free money market fund for liquid reserves, retired or higher taxable income investors wanting tax-free returns.	Excellent on long-term bonds (if interest rates decline). None on short-term money market instruments.	Normal risks associated with bonds, credit risk, interest rate risks, loss of purchasing power risk, risk of default, and so on.	Tax-free income may provide more spendable (after-tax) income.	Stick to high-grade bonds. Unit trusts are easier to sell if you need your money before maturity. Small issues are often expensive to sell. Because of inflation, tax-free municipal bonds have a history of being a bad long-term investment.
Annuities—fixed	Income grows tax-deferred. Issued by insurance companies.	Tax-deferred growth/guarantee of principal against loss, guaranteed minimum interest.	For conservative investors averse to risk. This conservative investment is a good alternative to taxable investments such as CDs, regular bonds, municipal bonds, and government bonds, etc.	None—you receive interest only on fixed annuities.	Risk of loss of purchasing power due to inflation, penalties if money is withdrawn prior to age 59½. TEFRA changes tax benefits substantially. Check out insurance company's financial strength.	Tax-free compound growth, guarantee of principal and interest.	Compare annuities. Understand loads or expenses, both from the insurance company and the potential tax liability caused by withdrawal of the money.

(Table 14-2 continues.)

(Table 14-2 continued.)

Investment	Description of Investment	Goal of Investment	Type of Investor	Potential for Growth	Primary Risk	Primary Reward	Notes
Oil and gas-completion financing	Partnership provides equipment and capital for completion of found reserves.	High cash flow that could increase or decrease depending upon the price of oil and gas.	Investor who believes that oil and gas business is a viable business and does not want speculative risks of drilling programs. For investors who want tax-sheltered cash flow.	Excellent	Very management intensive, risks of poor management decisions, risk of oil and gas price decline, risk of poor oil and gas reserves from completed well.	Tax-favored cash flow which would be substantial, inflation hedge.	Check out program and goals of specific program. For conservative individuals who wish good cash flow returns. Good opportunity for diversification.

From Financial and Investment Planning, Ltd., Suttons Bay, MI. With permission.

RECOMMENDED READING

Swanson R, & Swanson B: Tax Shelters: A Guide for Investors and Their Advisors. Homewood, IL, Dow-Jones/Erwin, 1985

Sommerfield RM: Federal Taxes and Management Decisions. Homewood, IL, Richard E. Erwin, Inc., 119833-1984

Porter, WT: The Touche Ross Guide to Personal Financial Management. Englewood Cliffs, NJ, Prentice-Hall, 1985

Tax Facts I/Tax Facts II. Cincinnati, OH: National Underwriter Co., 1986

Portfolio Management

To be successful, you, as an investor, must look at your investment assets as a portfolio. Specific goals and objectives should define categories of investments that will be utilized in your specific portfolio. Even that $2,000 that you stuck in your IRA account should be considered a portfolio. The decision-making process for construction of a portfolio should be the same for your IRA portfolio at $2,000 as it is for your pension portfolio at a half a million.

In portfolio construction, you first must define your goals. Figure 15-1 is a chart that we use in our practice for analyzing clients' specific goals and objectives for their portfolio. You should complete it to help yourself get an idea of your own investment constitution.

Once you have defined your goals, you must find the alternative methods of achieving that goal through specific investments and investment methods, and then you must make decisions regarding those investments and follow up on those decisions. Of course, on an ongoing basis, you should revise your decisions in the light of new information and specific developments that may affect your investments.

There are two specific methods (other than just randomly choosing an investment) that are used by investors to select specific investments. The first is the *fundamental* approach, and the second is the *technical* approach.

The fundamental approach stresses economic conditions such as level of employment, economic growth, financial conditions, and the level and direction of interest rates. If you are investing in common stocks, this approach may examine a company's earning capacity, its potential for growth, and its source for financing. The investment manager uses the fundamental approach to compare firms within an industry that he or she feels will produce superior investment results over time. The investment manager will try to identify those with the greatest potential and the strongest financial position. An emphasis is placed on a firm's economic performance and its potential to improve its position with its industry.

Ratios, financial data, and educated observations are the primary tools of the fundamental investment manager. The fundamental investment manager is often known as a basic value manager, or a bargain hunter. The fundamental investment manager is looking for investments based on

Date_____/_____/_____

FINANCIAL & INVESTMENT MANAGEMENT GROUP
PENSION SERVICE DESIGN, INC./FINANCIAL & INVESTMENT PLANNING LTD

PORTFOLIO ANALYSIS INFORMATION

Client/Investment Registration

_____

_____

_____

Type of Account: Taxable_____ Non-Taxable_____
What is your "goal" for your portfolio, i.e., high total return, stay ahead of inflation (maintain purchasing power), conservation of capital, etc.?

_____

In terms of your assets directed to investment areas, please rate how you feel about the following statements.

	Strongly Agree	Agree	Disagree	No Opinion
1-1) Short term safety of capital is very important				
1-2) Longer term safety of capital is very important				
2) Interested in pursuing growth investments, and willing to take the higher risks involved				
3) Income is very important				
4) A balanced program of income and growth investments makes the most sense				
5) A feel that hiring active, professional management which can "capitalize on opportunities and reduce risks" by using their knowledge, resources and experience to actively manage my portfolio makes the most sense to me				
6) Investments are cyclical and what may have been a great investment yesterday may not be good today. I feel my portfolio should be actively managed to take advantage of investment cycles				
7) Inflation protection (maintenance of purchasing power) is very important				

How much money would you want in a highly liquid state such as a savings account for emergency or opportunity reserve, terminations, retirements? $_____

I understand that all investments have risk, either "purchasing power risk" or "risk to principal".
Yes_____ No_____

I understand that retirement plan trusts have special tax status and that all dividends, capital gains, interest and other income grows tax free (therefore, a more "active" management style may be more beneficial than a "buy & hold" philosophy). Yes_____ No_____

Fig. 15-1.

120

some relative value approach, rather than based on a mania or the mass psychology or "flash" that a specific investment may have. Investment managers that manage under the fundamental approach often will buy a common stock, looking for performance over a 5 year or longer period. They will not be too concerned with the day-to-day fluctuations in asset values, but would rather be looking for favorable long-term total investment return. Many people like the idea of the fundamental approach to investment management; however, many individual investors cannot handle fluctuations in asset value.

Chapter 10 explains how to understand our cyclical economy, and a person who feels that there is merit and logic in the investment strategies described in Chapter 10 could call himself a fundamentalist, since these people would place strong emphasis on understanding the economic and business cycles that affect investments. These individuals may purchase an investment a little early in a cycle and, thus see some price decline. If they are strong in their convictions and accurate in their forecast, however, their specific investment decisions should bear bountiful fruit, although, perhaps over a long time frame.

In contrast to the fundamental analysis, technical analysis is the study of all factors related to the actual supply and demand of a specific investment through the use of charts and indicators that track the supply and demand. The technician will attempt to measure the "pulse of the market" and sometimes try to forecast future price movements.

A tremendous number of individual investors that use fundamental analysis to great success attest to the merits of the approach of fundamental analysis. However, technical analysis also must be considered valuable, ironically, because not all investors believe in it. A wise Wall Street observer once said "If everybody could buy at the bottom and sell at the top, the bottom would be the top and the top would be the bottom." The individual who understands both fundamental and technical analysis will know the strengths and weaknesses of each approach and should, therefore, have advantages on Wall Street.

There are many fine books on technical analysis and, just as fundamental analysis is an art and a science, technical analysis is also. Some of the nomenclature of a technician, or chartist as they are often called, are as follows: A technician will often look at charts (Bar Charts) that show a picture of an investments history. With a bar chart you can, with a glance, quickly see the stocks past actions and you can gain valuable perspective, especially if you contrast this with the fundamental approach, and overlay the different economic and business events that happened over that period, and analyze their effect on that specific investment.

There are several types of stock charts, such as a daily bar chart, that show the highest and lowest closing prices each day, as well as the number of shares traded daily. There are weekly bar charts, and there are also volume charts. Many national publications or daily newspapers will show the Dow Jones high/low close in bar chart form. By simply looking at these bar charts you can get a good feel for the market. For example, if there is a wide range between the high and the low for the day and the stock market closed very near the low, you can, by analyzing the specific events of that, perhaps get a good perspective on what the psychology is that is affecting the market at any given time.

A chartist will often look for specific patterns in a bar chart. Some of these patterns are called price support patterns, price resistant patterns, volume support, volume resistant, ascending triangles, descending triangles, inverse head and shoulder reversals, triple bottom reversals, etc.

At the end of this chapter there is a list of books that describe the technical methods of analysis, along with the fundamental methods of analysis in great detail. It is not the goal of this book to describe either of these approaches in great detail since the information on both of these approaches to investments would fill your family room bookshelves.

There are a few technical ratios and indicators that are very important to understand, as history has proved that they can be very good indicators of future events affecting the market.

The Dow Theory is one of the oldest and most famous technical tools of the stock market. It is used to forecast the future direction of the overall stock market, and uses the Dow Jones Industrial average and, occasionally, the Dow Jones Transportational averages as the guide. This theory is based on the observation that market movements are analogist to the movement of the sea, thus there are three movements in the market, all occurring simultaneously. Hourly or daily fluctuation, called ripples; secondary, or intermediate movements of 2 weeks to a month or more, called waves; and the primary trend, extending several months to a year or longer, called the tide, which is a primary trend and is generally referred to as a "bull" or "bear" market. Under this theory the daily fluctuations are of little value. Secondary movements must be closely watched as they can retrace one-third to two-thirds of the prior primary price change. The Dow Theory becomes very useful in the secondary movements to show new trends when the averages penetrate their previous secondary peaks.

Another technical indicator is the short interest ratio. This ratio is a contrary indicator of the market on the whole. Short sellers sell shares that they don't own that must be purchased later, they hope, at lower prices (for the investor). A large short interest ratio indicates that many investors anticipate lower prices. It also represents potential buying power. In the past, short interest ratio has been a reliable market indicator. The short interest ratio recently has become distorted because many investors use stock options and futures as alternative methods of selling short during bear markets. It can, however, be a very good contrary indicator, generally when the short interest ratio is between 1 and 1.6 it is regarded as neutral, and a ratio of more than 1.6 is "bullish." This has generally been a very good time to buy stocks—when the short interest has been at least double the average daily volume, i.e., when the ratio is 2 or more.

It is the widely accepted rule on Wall Street that the odd lot small investor (which is a buyer or seller of less than 100 shares) is usually wrong. The odd lot ratio can be used at moments of extreme optimism and extreme pessimism. It, historically, has not been a good indicator during periods other than this, however, it is good to consider odd lot short sales and total off lot sales. (The short interest ratio is calculated by dividing the New York Stock Exchange short interest total by the average daily New York Stock Exchange volume over the same period.)

Are there stock market cycles? Some analysts think so. It is interesting to note that except for one incident, every fourth year since 1914 has been a good time to buy stocks. Moreover, every fifth year since 1905 has been a year of rising stock prices.

When choosing specific investments for construction of your portfolio, it is very important that you understand both the fundamental approach in analyzing the investment value and the technical approach. The technical approach is very good at pointing out the forces of market psychology, and helping you to predict human nature. When combined with the fundamental approach it makes it very easy to see whether an investment is going to mania (either to become substantially overvalued and, thus, makes it either a sell opportunity or, undervalued and a substantial buy opportunity).

A good example of a portfolio manager in action is the following taken from a brochure describing what a very successful manager looks at when choosing stocks for his or her client portfolios.

Earnings Growth

The company must demonstrate sustained earnings growth. Earnings from continuing operations should have doubled in the last 10 years. The quality of earnings, based on conservative accounting practices, is an important factor. Confidence in earnings predictability also is important.

Dividend Stability

The dividend must not have been cut more than once in the last 10 years. Dividends that are consistent and that increase regularly are given preference in weighting. This demonstrates management's ability to handle cash flow and earnings for the benefit of shareholders.

Low Price/Earnings Multiple

The stock's price to earnings multiple should be less than the market's general multiple. This provides the opportunity for multiple expansion. A low multiple prevents the purchase of stock that could have considerable risk if earnings contract.

Discount to Book Value

The stock should be selling below its tangible book value per share. (Tangible book value is equal to total assets minus all liabilities and good will.) Changes in earnings and price/earnings ratios can be sudden and violent. However, changes in book value are more gradual. Book value represents an intrinsic value that is more representative of the worth of the company than its daily price quotation.

High Liquidity

The company's current assets less current liabilities and long-term debt, per share, should be high in relation to the price of the stock.

Financial Soundness

The long-term debt should be less than 40 percent of the total capitalization. During difficult periods, a company's cash flow should be directed to investments in operations rather than interest expense. A highly leveraged balance sheet can become a hindrance to performance and financial soundness.

Quality Management

The company should be run by capable and honest management with a history of being reasonable with and fair to all shareholders.

Shareholder

Ownership of the stock should be weighted towards insiders and away from institutions. We want management and directors to have their personal wealth invested in the company and its performance. We prefer companies shrinking their capitalization through the repurchase of stock and the reduction of debt.

Hidden Assets

Assets that are not on the balance sheet are considered additional value. Hidden assets such as a LIFE reserve, high appraised value, understated natural resource assets, or an over-funded pension plan can significantly add to shareholder net worth.

High Cash Flow

Cash flow per share should considerably higher than earnings per share. It has been demonstrated that strong cash flow allows a company to generate greater wealth over the long term. Debt does not need to be added as quickly, if at all, for expansion or reinvestment. A high discretionary cash flow, after capital expenditures and dividends, is very attractive.

Chart Pattern

Technical analysis should indicate that a stock is presently attractive for investing without undue speculation. Chart patterns show the history of a stock's price and the volume of its trading at various levels. We typically seek "bases" in a stock's patterns on the belief that speculators will not own the stock or be interested in it at that moment. Reading the chart of a stock is often an art, but in today's market it is a necessary skill to complement our fundamental analysis.

Potential for Favorable Development

There are always undervalued common stocks. To maximize total return for our shareholders the fund not only looks for undervalued securities, but anticipates events that will close the gap between the stock's price and intrinsic value. Such an event may be the company repurchasing a sizable number of outstanding shares, increased merger activity within their industry, new products, or the redeployment of assets.

> Value Investing for the '80's
> The Milwaukee Company
> 250 East Wisconsin Avenue
> Milwaukee, WI 53202

RECOMMENDED READING

Smith, Charles W: The Mind of the Market. Rowan and Littlefield, Totowe, NJ, 1981

Dreman, David: The New Contrarian Investment Strategy. Random House, New York, 1980, 1982

Schulz, James: The Economics of Aging. Wadsworth Printing Company, 1980

Ghman, Lawrence and Joehnk, Michael: Fundamentals of Investing. Harper-Row, New York, 1981

Ping, Martin J: Technical Analysis Explained. McGraw-Hill Books, New York, 1980

16

The Long-term Diversified
Portfolio Strategy

You have learned in other chapters that there is no investment that is always the best, nor is there is an investment management style that works in every investment cycle. However, many investors are always looking for investment techniques that are "best" in any investment cycle. The fact is, you should not look for the "best" investment but rather look for a strategy or portfolio structure designed to win the favorable long-term investment performance game.

Naturally you can use a rear view mirror approach and manage your portfolio by using the investments that have performed well in the past. Making an investment based purely on the past, however, can prove to be foolhardy and cause the purchasing of assets that may be substantially overvalued because of a mania. (As learned earlier, a mania is when an investment becomes either substantially overvalued or substantially undervalued because of an euphoria about its value.) In spite of the fact that most assets go to mania—such as when interest rates went up to 20 percent and the stock market crashed in the 1973/1974 cycle—history shows that certain assets, over time, perform substantially better than other assets. For example, common stocks as a class of assets have substantially out-performed most other classes of assets over nearly every (or any) 25-year period since the turn of the century, and small company common stocks as a class of assets have done even better.

History also tells us that real estate investments have substantially out-performed investments such as CDs and short- and long-term government and corporate bonds through moderate and rapid inflationary periods. Table 11-1 (see page 88) illustrates how certain classes of assets have performed over time during different economic environments. Making educated investment choices will also enhance your investment performance on most assets, such as using professionally managed mutual funds when investing in common stocks or bonds. Thus, if you have a choice of having a portfolio diversified among, for example, the Standard and Poor's 500 stocks, which is an unmanaged proxy of stocks, over having an individual

127

choose specific stocks from that pool of assets, history has shown that a skillful portfolio manager will have had superior results. The investment specialist would, because it appears that oil prices might decline, choose to exclude oil stocks in his or her portfolio, and instead, purchase stocks in companies such as airlines and other transportation companies that would benefit from declining oil prices.

Most money managers do not like to admit that they are not consistently able to always choose winning assets. Most good money managers have, over time, however, been able to tip the scales in favor of out-performing asset classes as a whole. These managers won't win every investment game by always choosing the winning asset for that year; however, many are able to consistently turn out favorable seasons. Thus, to develop a top-notch portfolio you must take a common sense, long-term view and properly diversify your holdings.

The long-term diversified portfolio strategy is designed for the patient pragmatic investor who has a desire to have favorable, consistent total returns over the long term. The long-term portfolio strategy is designed to diversify out the risk of each asset class while still taking advantage of professional managers who have consistently out-performed unmanaged assets. This portfolio strategy is not designed to make an individual rich over night, but is designed for the investor who can think long term and, as stated in Chapter 13, understands that all investments have risk, either inflation/loss of purchasing power risk or loss of principal risk.

To develop a top-notch long-term diversified strategy five key elements must be addressed to help assure investment results. They are as follows:

1. Diversify your portfolio by class of investment (or asset type). Diversify those assets by date of maturity, predictability of return, and diversify within each class of investment. For example, if you are going to have 20 percent of your portfolio in common stocks, do not put that 20 percent in one individual common stock, but rather you should have at least 20 different individual common stocks, or better yet purchase common stock mutual funds which have built-in diversification.
2. Always have at least some money in each type of asset, even if it is only a small percent of your total portfolio.
3. Always choose the best advisors to manage the assets of each category, such as choosing a good common stock fund manager. However, on assets that are more passive such as government bonds or money market instruments, minimize commissions, sales, and management fees, as much as possible. In addition, always diversify among money managers. This is very easy and can be done even with a $1,000 IRA portfolio through mutual funds. No front-end load mutual fund charges a $250 investor, as a percentage of assets, no more than a $1,000,000 investor would be charged. Mutual funds are a great bargain for the small investor.

4. Slowly, over 3 months to 1 year, dollar cost average into assets such as common stocks if they appear overvalued. When in doubt as to whether an asset is overvalued, you should dollar cost average into that asset.

5. Take profits on assets to keep your percentages in line with your original portfolio weighting goals. If an asset category loses values, so that it is behind its original goal, take the dividends from your other assets to get the weighting up on that particular asset. This disciplined approach helps you to purchase assets when they are undervalued while forcing you to sell assets as they become overvalued.

Figures 16-1 and 16-2 illustrate a long-term diversified strategy in actual practice to achieve various investment goals. Figure 16-3 is a worksheet to use to develop your own long-term diversified strategy. Figures 16-4 and 16-1 are portfolios that try to provide predictability of returns. Figure 16-4 provides predictability of income and Figure 16-1 predictability of principal. The businessperson's risk strategy (Fig. 16-2) is for the investor who is more patient and long-term oriented than the investor who wants short-term predictability, at the expense of long-term results.

Notice that even the investor seeking short-term predictability has common stocks, gold, international stocks and bonds in his or her portfolio, to help offset inflation and to get favorable long term results. In addition, notice the investor that wants shorter term predictability has more assets that are actively managed. The reason for active management is that even longer term government bonds, etc., will fluctuate in value, depending upon the interest rate cycle as learned in an earlier chapter.

If managers feel that interest rates are going to rise, they will move their clients into shorter maturity bonds, while if they feel interest rates are going to be stable or are trending down, they will move their clients into longer term bonds. Notice, however, that in spite of this, we still have longer term bonds (that are just bought and held) because even the best manager may miss a cycle.

Most of the core holdings are designed to give fairly predictable returns. These help to balance out the portfolio and reduce the risks inherent in the assets that are more longer term oriented such as common stocks, gold, and international investments. Understand that the aforementioned investments should, and most probably will, have substantially greater returns than your core holdings because they have more risk. Thus, by changing your percentages you can control your portfolio risk. Most assets however, should be actively managed either through purchasing a good, well managed mutual fund, or hiring a good money manager who has expertise in managing that class of assets. The core holdings generally should not be actively managed but rather passively managed, often through using no-load mutual funds. Mutual funds are usually cheaper then purchasing individual bonds or CDs, etc. because of the economy of size.

THE LONG-TERM DIVERSIFIED STRATEGY
Sample Portfolio Strategy to Provide Income
(Predictability of Income)

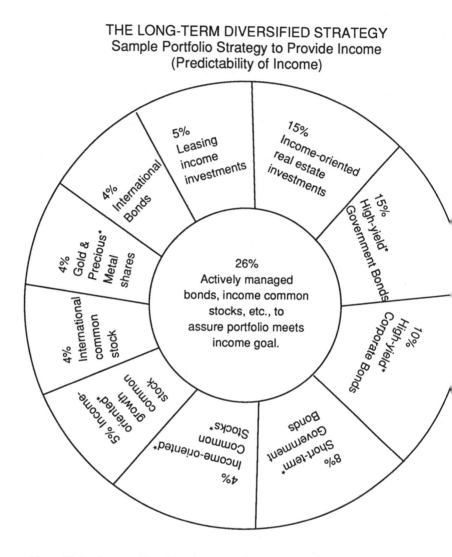

Note: If the Income Portfolio is to provide a stated income goal, i.e., $7000 a year income on a $100,000 portfolio, your portfolio should generate enough income to provide for that goal.

When developing a Retirement Income Portfolio, you must expect to live forever and thus, your portfolio should grow in size to offset inflation. A goal of 6% to 7% income and 4% to 6% capital growth is reasonable.

Fig. 16-1. Sample portfolio strategy to provide income.

THE LONG-TERM DIVERSIFIED STRATEGY
Sample "Predictability of Capital" Strategy
(Emphasis on Capital Preservation)

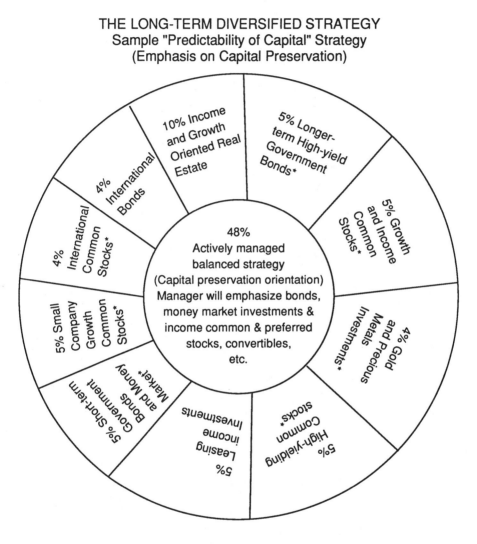

Note: Core assets should be managed to take advantage of cycles--other assets should also be managed through the use of no or low-load mutual funds with good managers.

*Generally purchased through a professionally managed no or low-load mutual fund or common trust. (It is better to over-diversify than under-diversify.)

Fig. 16-2. Sample "predictability of capital" strategy. (From Financial & Investment Planning, Ltd., Suttons Bay, MI. With permission.)

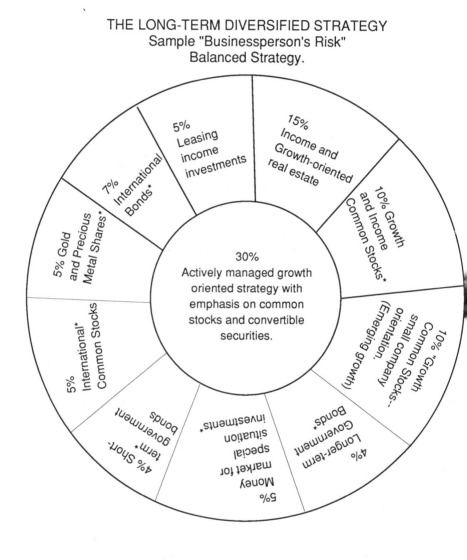

Fig. 16-3. Sample "businessperson's risk" balanced strategy. (From Financial & Investment Planning, Ltd., Suttons Bay, MI. With permission.)

PORTFOLIO STRUCTURE WORKSHEET

Investment Goals: _____
(Examples: capital preservation, growth in capital, balanced strategy, provide retirement income, etc.)

_____% Short term government bonds, CDs, money market instruments.

_____% High yielding longer term government bonds.

_____% High yielding longer term corporate bonds.

_____% Income and growth, "equity" common stock in investments such as: income common stocks, convertable and preferred common stocks, convertable bonds.

_____% Growth common stock investments (smaller company and emerging growth security).

_____% Gold and precious metals investments.

_____% International common stocks.

_____% International common bonds.

_____% Real Estate.

_____% Leasing income investments.

_____% Actively managed portfolio with emphasis on: (1) growth, (2) growth/ income or balanced strategy, (3) income orientation, etc.—managed to take advantage of investment cycles.

Note: Your portfolio should have at least some of each of the above investments in it, even if the percentage is on 2% to 4%. Review your portfolio structure often but change it slowly other than the actively managed portion and the reinvestment of income.

Fig. 16-4. The long-term diversified strategy. (From Financial & Investment Planning, Ltd., Suttons Bay, MI. With permission.)

When purchasing real estate use real estate investment trusts, participating mortgage limited partnerships, and real estate partnerships that are designed to produce income. Income real estate partnerships generally buy commercial buildings and lease them back to major tenants. They provide returns from two sources; the income from the leases and, hopefully, appreciation in the underlying real estate value. Growth real estate programs (generally housing limited partnerships or perhaps raw land), produce very little in the way of income return, with returns coming from growth of the underlying asset values.

One of the biggest problems with a well diversified approach is bookkeeping. However, there are a number of trust companies throughout the United States that will manage self-directed trusts under a flat fee system where they do not charge an asset fee. They will let you diversify among assets, perhaps having only a transaction charge or a flat fee for each portfolio.

Using the long-term strategy allows you to spend your money where it should be spent, on very good common stock money managers. This will help because you can pay very low fees or commissions on your core holdings. It liberates you to put your money where your investment management dollars should go, which is the common stock and bond element of your portfolio.

You will often find that when you hire a manager to manage your whole portfolio he or she may use a strategy similar to the long-term strategy, however, you are paying for management of core holdings that are really not actively managed, such as shorter and longer term government and corporate bonds, gold, or international investments. These investments typically are purchased to help diversify out some of the risks of the other assets in the portfolio, i.e., small company common stocks,etc. It is unnecessary to pay a money manager to manage these assets especially when in reality he or she may not be managing these assets, and is just using them to control risk.

It is advisable to sit down with a good money manager periodically to go over your portfolio to decide which assets should be managed and which assets should be core holdings and not managed. Also you could hire a manager for a fee or call up the mutual fund manager to discuss your portfolio with him or her, or get a few newsletters that will help educate yourself, and then you can informally manage your core holdings. Some investment professionals will manage your core holdings without charging an ongoing asset fee if they get the commissions generated from those assets and/or if their firm receives the fees for managing the actively managed holdings.

It is better to be over-diversified than under-diversified in your holdings. However, the diversification must be proper and thus, you should have many different classes of assets with many different maturities and/or names of assets in each portfolio. For example, if you are going to be investing 10 percent in real estate (which may be a small dollar amount) it is better to purchase a diversified limited partnership or a real estate investment trust rather than going out and buying one piece of raw land south of town, because you have an undiversified risk in that one real estate holding.

If you see a special situation, it would be appropriate to allocate 5 or 10 percent of your portfolio for the purpose of speculating or investing in special situations that you feel would be proper, however, you still should have some diversification within that asset category and not consider that asset exclusively for that particular category.

Most investors fail because they get drawn into manias. One of the key benefits of the long-term portfolio strategy is that it helps you to avoid the manias because when an asset becomes overvalued, you will have a tendency to sell those assets during the mania to keep the proper percentage in that asset. As an asset becomes substantially undervalued, the portfolio strategy will help you to purchase more assets of that category to get the weighting back up to assure proper diversification. Selling profitable assets and buying unprofitable assets is often very difficult, but the long-term portfolio strategy helps to disciple you to do this.

If you are after spectacular returns, the long-term portfolio strategy may not be for you. If you are after consistent, somewhat predictable longer term performance, then you should strongly consider using this approach for your own investments.

It is interesting to note that with this strategy, if 90 percent of your portfolio averages 10 percent, and 10 percent averages 30 percent, your overall portfolio return would be 12 percent. Thus, even though you could invest 90 percent of your portfolio in more conservative assets, the 10 percent of your invested assets toward superior returns (i.e., small company common stocks, international investments, and real estate, etc.) could have such favorable performance over the long term, to make you very happy.

When choosing specific assets for the categories in your portfolio you should look at each asset as diligently as if that particular asset were making up 100 percent of your portfolio. Carefully analyze each of the assets and categories and the different methodologies of investment that you could use in each asset category, and then choose the best manager. For example, if you are going to put 10 percent of your portfolio into a small company's common stock mutual funds, choose mutual funds that have managers who have had excellent, long-term results. "Go with the winner" when you choose mutual funds. Make sure when choosing mutual funds that the manager who gave the fund that spectacular performance is still managing that fund. Stick to the mutual funds (especially for small company common stock funds) that have a small amount of assets representing their portfolio, i.e., under four hundred million dollars in total assets, because you want each of the small company common stocks that portfolio manager chooses, to be able to have significant impact on the fund portfolio. If the fund gets too large, it becomes unresponsive, like trying to stop or turn a cruise liner.

With bond mutual funds, choose a large, well diversified fund. For balanced funds the need for a small asset base is not as important.

When choosing the real estate or leasing portions of your portfolio, try to go with managers that have proven track records. Try to go with portfolios (especially with real estate) that are specified so you know exactly what the investments are that will make up your portfolio. Try to avoid blind pools. Also, if you are buying partnerships for the real estate portion of your portfolio, have a bias towards purchasing partnerships that are on the resale or secondary market to avoid the start-up fees, commissions, and expenses that can be substantial for some partnerships. Today there are partnerships and real estate investment trusts that have low, or greatly reduced, loads that are very suitable for most portfolios.

This long-term diversified strategy is not just for the big investor. It works as well for a $2,000 Individual Retirement Account (IRA) portfolio as it does for the million dollar pension portfolio (although an IRA portfolio of $2,000 would have trouble purchasing all the different assets).

As mentioned previously, you should monitor your portfolio at least on a quarterly basis and reevaluate the asset weightings on a semi-annual or annual basis, to make sure your portfolio is performing favorably. However, have patience with your portfolio and your managers, which means allow them 2 or 3 years to show you their stuff, rather than firing them after the first quarter. The long-term investment strategy is for the mature long-term oriented investor, so don't hire your managers and then put restrictions on them that make them feel that if they don't perform in the first quarter you are going to fire them. This would be counter-productive, because rather than committing your assets as they feel for best long-term performance, they may default to putting substantially all your assets into asset categories that produce predictable returns, thus defeating the purpose of the long-term diversified portfolio strategy.

This portfolio strategy can work very well for someone that is retired; however, the weighting should be changed in favor of providing sufficient yield to live on (see Fig. 16-1). For example, if the portfolio is $100,000 and you feel you need $9,000 a year in income from the portfolio, the $9,000 in dividends, cash flow, or interest should be generated predictably from the assets in the portfolio. In today's marketplace, leasing investments, income real estate programs, and corporate and long-term government bonds do provide substantial amounts of income, while the other portfolio assets would be oriented towards offsetting inflation. Through changes in the asset weighting, you should be able to get a portfolio that will successfully meet your income goals, while also having your capital increased to help offset inflation.

As with any investment strategy there are no guarantees that this diversified approach will work. History shows, however, that favorable returns should result through investments in a portfolio structured under this methodology. Naturally, the weighting should change in your portfolio as we move into new economic cycles. During inflationary periods you would have less in fixed income investments, such as government and corporate bonds. During noninflationary periods, or periods of lower inflation, you should have a heavier weighting towards bonds. Remember, the key to this strategy is *diversify*.

RECOMMENDED READING

Little JB, Rhodes L: Understanding Wall Street. Library Publishing Company, Cockeysvill, MD,1978

Gipson J: Winning the Investment Game A Guide for all Seasons. Mc-Graw-Hill Books, New York, 1984

Mayo H: Investments. Dryden Press, Hinsdale, IL,1983

17

Retirement Planning (working when you want, if you want, how you want, and where you want)

Tax favored retirement plan trusts are the most efficient method of accumulating wealth. However, many physicians underutilize retirement plan trusts because they are unaware of the flexibility and financial speed a retirement plan trust can add to the attainment of their goals. Retirement plan trusts can be used to create wealth and build net worth for reasons such as education of children, buying a second home, financial security, and, naturally, retirement. This chapter will deal with accumulating wealth through utilizing and understanding the tools and techniques of retirement plans.

The wealth-creating efficiency of retirement plans comes from three distinct sources:

1. The value of the current tax deduction allowed on contributions to the retirement plan.
2. The value of accumulating earnings on the retirement plan trust's investments tax deferred.
3. The comparative advantage of utilizing tax qualified retirement plans as a wealth accumulator when compared to other investments or wealth creation strategies.

Table 17-1 illustrates the pension or IRA break-even holding period. This table shows the comparative advantage of getting a current deduction and compound tax-free growth on a retirement plan trust, compared to investing the money in a taxable account without the benefits of the current tax deduction and tax deferred growth on retirement plans.

Thus, if you were in a 30 percent tax bracket and earned 11 percent on your investment in your IRA or pension, or in your taxable account, and you were to cash in your IRA or pension after 4.28 years you would be ahead over not using a retirement plan and paying the taxes. If you have

139

Table 17-1
Pension or IRA Breakeven Holding Periods

Average annual yield to withdrawal*
(Includes 10% penalty for distribution made prior to 59 ½)

Constant Marginal tax rate (%)*	6%	7%	8%	9%	10%	11%	12%	13%	14%	15%	16%	17%
10	19.63	16.83	14.72	13.09	11.78	10.71	9.82	9.06	8.41	7.85	7.36	6.93
15	13.91	11.92	10.43	9.27	8.34	7.59	6.95	6.42	5.96	5.56	5.22	4.91
20	11.13	9.54	8.35	7.42	6.68	6.07	5.56	5.14	4.77	4.45	4.17	3.93
25	9.54	8.18	7.16	6.36	5.72	5.20	4.77	4.40	4.09	3.82	3.58	3.37
30	8.56	7.34	6.42	5.71	5.14	4.67	4.28	3.95	3.67	3.43	3.21	3.02
35	7.96	6.82	5.97	5.30	4.77	4.34	3.98	3.67	3.41	3.18	2.98	2.81
40	7.60	6.51	5.70	5.06	4.56	4.14	3.80	3.51	3.26	3.04	2.85	2.68
45	7.43	6.37	5.57	4.95	4.46	4.05	3.72	3.43	3.19	2.97	2.79	2.62
50	7.44	6.38	4.48	4.96	4.46	4.06	3.72	3.43	3.19	2.98	2.79	2.63

*Rates are continuously compounded for both taxes and average annual yield. Rates not continuously compounded can be substituted for a rough idea of the breakeven point. Example: 30% tax bracket - 12% yield = 4.28 years for breakeven.
From Pension Service Design, Inc. Suttons Bay, MI. With permission.

children that you need to educate and they are four years from college and you are in a 30 percent tax bracket and feel comfortable earning 11 percent or greater on your retirement plan trust, this might be the most efficient method of accumulating wealth for that future need.

Figure 17-1 illustrates in numerical and graphic form the tremendous advantage that a retirement plan has over the alternative taxable investment program. Assuming the $10,000 outlay, a 30 percent tax bracket and 12 percent investment return, after 20 years the taxable account will grow to $286,967, and you can quickly see that even if you cashed in your retirement plan (approximately $572,749) and paid 30 percent of that in taxes ($171,824), that you would have more money ($400,924 compared to $286,907) than you would under a taxable scheme. If you combine the tax favored aspects to the magic of compound returns, you will quickly realize that everyone should retire rich, if they will utilize the tax favored retirement plans to their maximum advantage. Everyone should try to save at least 10 percent of their earnings in a retirement plan. If they can do this, it will grow tax free and substantial wealth can be created.

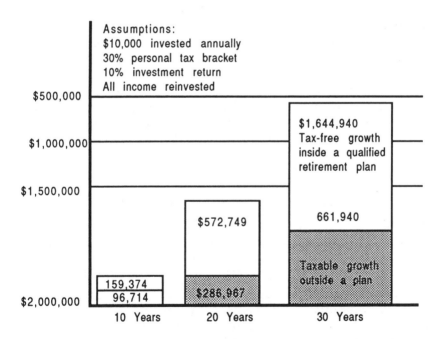

Note: Taxable growth figures assume $10,000 annual investment with $3,000 paid in taxes for a net contribution of $7,000 and a taxable 10% yield or 7% after tax yield.

Fig. 17-1. Wealth accumulation and tax benefits of a retirement plan. From Pension Service Design, Inc., Suttons Bay, MI. With permission.

The average physician makes about $92,000 per year and Table 17-2 illustrates funding of a retirement plan with a $10,000 annual contribution. If you are in a 30 percent tax bracket and you put $10,000 annually into a retirement plan, the net cost is only $7,000, making the net after tax effect of putting $10,000 per year away, roughly 8 percent of the average physician's income. Naturally, 10 percent of income should be a minimum goal and you should put substantially more in if you want to retire earlier than age 65, are close to retirement, or if you have other financial goals that you want to address (such as accumulating wealth for children's education, etc.). Table 17-2 illustrates the magic of compound returns and the importance of favorable compound returns on your retirement fund. Assuming a $10,000 annual contribution, over 35 years the difference between 12 and 15 percent compound return yields 100 percent greater benefit, although the additional return was only 25 percent of the 12 percent (i.e., 3 percent).

Because of inflation's impact on retirement plans, it is very important that you get in your mind the goals of setting aside a certain percentage of your salary or income annually rather than a fixed amount of dollars to help offset the effects of inflation. Table 17-3 illustrates inflation's effect on a pension fund value of $1,000,000 in today's dollars. The best way to offset inflation is to set aside a certain percentage of your income. Thus, as your income goes up, the percentage that you are putting into your retirement plan will also go up.

Clients ask me how much money they should save for retirement. I usually tell them all that they can afford, consistent with maintaining their present lifestyle. Depending on their age and specific circumstances, we may try to put in a minimum of $500 monthly into a retirement plan, to

Table 17-2

Everyone Should Retire Rich: The Importance of Favorable Compound Return in Your Pension Fund—$10,000. Annual Contribution

Years to Retirement	5% Compound Return	10% Compound Return	12% Compound Return	15% Compound Return
05	$ 58,019.	$ 67,156.	$ 71,152.	$ 77,537.
10	132,068.	175,312.	196,546.	233,493.
15	226,575.	349,497.	417,533.	547,175.
20	342,183.	630,025.	806,987.	1,178,101.
25	501,135.	1,081,818.	1,493,339.	2,447,120.
30	697,608.	1,809,434.	2,702,926.	4,999,569.
35	948,383.	2,981,268.	4,834,631.	10,133,457.

From Pension Service Design, Inc. Suttons Bay, MI. With permission.

Table 17-3
Inflation Effects on Your Pension Fund—The Value of $1,000,000
in Today's Purchasing Power at Various Rates of Inflation

End of Year	5%	8%	10%	14%
05	$ 783,530.	$ 680,580.	$ 620,920.	$ 519,370.
10	613,910.	463,190.	385,540.	269,740.
15	481,020.	315,240.	239,390.	140,100.
25	295,300.	146,020.	92,300	37,790.
35	181,290.	67,630.	35,580.	10,190.

From Pension Service Design, Inc., Suttons Bay, MI. With permission.

ensure that there will at least be a basic amount of money accumulating towards retirement. Thus, you should be able to tell by now that the keys to wealth at retirement are:

1. Saving a percentage of your income
2. Trying to start early
3. Utilizing tax favored retirement plan trusts
4. Using proper investments, as described in Chapters 10 through 16.

In summary, retirement plans have three primary tax advantages:

1. All contributions to the retirement plan within the IRS limits are 100 percent tax deductible
2. All earnings in the retirement plan trust grow tax free
3. At retirement or distribution, there may be special tax advantages.

DESIGNING A RETIREMENT TAX SHELTER THAT FITS

Once you have decided that it makes sense to have a retirement plan to help accumulate wealth, the most important decision is the design of your plan. It should be designed for maximum efficiency and it should be designed specifically to your goals. All retirement plans have certain limitations and specific characteristics that will affect your situation. Thus, you must understand the proper priorities in retirement planning.

Your number one priority in retirement planning should be to fund your personal IRA, and secondly, your spouse's IRA, since funding your IRA is very simple and does not require any contribution for your employees. Also, funding of IRAs does not require the filing of annual forms and trust documents with the IRS, is simple to set up and maintain, and has low costs. If your spouse is not working, put him or her on salary at $2,000 a year, and put that $2,000 a year into a retirement plan on their behalf.

If you want to fund more than your IRA, the qualified retirement plan you should first consider is a profit sharing plan and whether it will fulfill your needs and goals. Second, you should consider a money purchase plan, and third, a defined benefit plan. Table 17-4 explains the different characteristics and limitations on the different retirement plan types; use Table 17-4 in helping you decide the best type of retirement plan for you.

In setting up a qualified retirement plan, as an employer you must make decisions as to: who will be covered; under what conditions the employees will be eligible for participation; what benefits your employees will receive upon retirement, death, disability, and severance of employment; how they will receive their benefits; and whether the employee will contribute toward the cost of these benefits. Naturally, legal requirements and IRS limitations create many limitations in the design of a plan. Basically, employees must be covered if they work for you over 1000 hours a year; are over age 21; and work for you or for a company that you own or in which you have a substantial interest. The plan must not discriminate in any way in favor of officers, shareholders, or highly compensated employees that are often called the "prohibitive group." This does not mean that your employees will receive the same amount of money that you put in on your own behalf; it just means that the plan cannot discriminate in favor of this group. The IRS has specific guidelines for retirement plans that, if not violated, will generally be accepted by them as not being discriminatory.

The primary way to beef-up contributions for yourself is to integrate the plan based on social security. The IRS allows employers to design a plan that reduces the contributions for lower paid employees based on the amount of contribution that you made on their behalf to the social security system. This also works on the defined benefit system. Table 17-5 illustrates the utilization of integration on plans, both profit sharing/money purchase and defined benefit plans. Note how the use of proper integration can reduce substantially the contributions for lower paid employees. Thus, if you have a large staff, by integrating your retirement plan you can reduce the cost of covering your employees, while still putting a substantial amount of money away for yourself.

In setting up your retirement plan you are going to need to employ the services of a pension consultant who can advise you on the nuances of the retirement plans and also design a plan specifically for your needs. There are many very fine consulting firms throughout the country, and your accountant or attorney should be able to refer you to one. In our office we have a strong partiality towards using prototype retirement plans for money purchase and profit sharing plans since the costs of establishing a prototype plan are much less than they are to have custom documents. Also, prototype plans can have tremendous flexibility and are easy to amend, all of which keeps the cost of the annual administration on the retirement plan small.

Table 17-4

Retirement Plan Types

Type of Plan	Key Characteristics	Maximum Allowable Contribution	Can Plan be Integrated?	Benefits and Advantages of Plan	Disadvantages of Plan	Set up Deadline	Contribution Deadline
Profit-sharing (defined contribution plan).	Flexibility, simplicity. Forfeitures are reallocated to remaining participants (within limits).	15 % of salary; maximum contribution per participant is $30,000. With possible adjustments for inflation in future.	Yes	Simple to administer and explain. Favors younger employees. Forfeitures reallocated. Usually contributions must be 3% of all eligible employees salary.	Limits on contributions. Benefits often are not significant for older employees.	End of fiscal year. For self-employed individuals, end of calendar year.	Date of filing federal tax return, including extensions, for contributions based on previous year's compensation.
Money purchase plan (defined contribution plan).	Simplest type of pension plan. Employer contributions are fixed as a percentage of eligible payroll. Often used in tandem with a profit-sharing plan.	For corporate plans, 25% of salary. Maximum contribution per participant is $30,000. For self-employed, 20% of gross salary, or 25% of net salary. With possible adjustments for inflation in future.	Yes	Larger contribution than profit-sharing plan. Simple to administer and explain. Favors younger employees.	Contributions are required. Benefits often are not significant for older employees.	End of fiscal year. For self-employed individuals, end of calendar year.	Date of filing federal tax return, including extensions, for contributions based on previous year's compensation.
Defined benefit plan	Benefits are defined in advance. Contributions can be substantial. Provides employees with a predictable retirement income.	No limits on contributions. Contributions must be adequate to provide stated benefit. Benefit cannot be over $90,000 a year. With possible adjustments for inflation in future.	Yes	Substantial contributions allowed for older employees. Plans are great wealth accumulators. They function well with a good actuary and proper administration.	Complexity. Plans are more sophisticated than defined contribution plans. Contributions are fixed. Administrative costs are generally higher.	End of fiscal year. For self-employed individuals, end of calendar year.	Date of filing federal tax return, including extensions, for contributions based on previous year's compensation.

(Table 17-4 continues.)

145

(Table 17-4 continued.)

Type of Plan	Key Characteristics	Maximum Allowable Contribution	Can Plan be Integrated?	Benefits and Advantages of Plan	Disadvantages of Plan	Set up Deadline	Contribution Deadline
Simplified Employer Pension Plan (SEP IRA)	A form of IRA with higher maximum contributions. Simple to administer (no government reporting required).	15% of contribution, but not more than $15,000 annually per participant. (only first $200,000 of compensation may be used to determine percentage of contribution).	Yes	Flexibility. Contributions are tax-deductible. Earnings grown tax-free. Can be set up after year-end (until April 15) for contribution based on prior year's compensation.	Limits on contributions. Does not have same tax advantages as corporate plans do at retirement, death, or disability. Cannot retire prior to age 59½ without substantial 10% tax penalty.	April 15	April 15
Individual Retirement Account (IRA)	Flexibility. All wage earners qualify for an IRA. Does not have to cover employees. See "IRA Facts" (p. 150).	$2,000 or 100% of income. $2,250 if non-working spouse included.	Yes	Simplicity. Can be in tandem with other retirement plans.	Contribution limitations make benefits less significant than those provided by other retirement plans.	April 15 or prior to filing tax return, including extension.	April 15 or prior to filing tax return, including extension.
6% voluntary non-deductible contributions to qualified retirement plans.	Better than non-deductible IRA because you can take up to 6% of your salary and contribute it to your pension plan or profit-sharing plan and it will grow tax deferred.	6% of salary not to exceed $30,000 including contributions to plan.	Yes	Grow tax free—you can take your money out at any time at no tax cost as long as you leave all your growth in plan. Great for college education etc., or anything you want prior to age 59½		Can be added as adoption on any qualified retirement plan at any time.	N/A—Since contributions are non-deductible, it really does not have a deadline "per se."

From Pension Service Design, Inc. Suttons Bay, MI. With permission.

Table 17-5
Comparison of Plans

Age	Income	Oversimplified Contribution to Integrated Profit Sharing Plan— 9.3% of 1st $15,000. 15% of Excess	Oversimplified Maximum Contribution to Profit Sharing Plan	Oversimplified Maximum Contribution to Tandem 10% Money Purchase Plan with 15% Profit Sharing Plan	Contribution To Maximum Defined Benefit Plan Assuming 7% Assumption	Value of Defined Benefit Plan Assets at Age 65 (Funding Goal)
60	$100,000.	$14,145.	$15,000.	$25,000.	$134,753.	$1,031,400.
55	100,000.	14,145.	15,000.	25,000.	61,071.	1,031,400.
50	100,000.	14,145.	15,000.	25,000.	34,564.	1,031,400.
45	100,000.	14,145.	15,000.	25,000.	21,485.	1,031,400.
40	100,000.	14,145.	15,000.	25,000.	14,036.	1,031,400.
35	100,000.	14,145.	15,000.	25,000.	9,443.	1,031,400.
30	100,000.	14,145.	15,000.	25,000.	6,473.	1,031,400.
25	100,000.	14,145.	15,000.	25,000.	4,492.	1,031,400.
60	15,000.	1,395.	2,250.	3,750.	22,459.	171,900.
55	15,000.	1,395.	2,250.	3,750.	10,179.	171,900.
50	15,000.	1,395.	2,250.	3,750.	5,761.	171,900.
45	15,000.	1,395.	2,250.	3,750.	3,581.	171,900.
40	15,000.	1,395.	2,250.	3,750.	2,339.	171,900.
35	15,000.	1,395.	2,250.	3,750.	1,574.	171,900.
30	15,000.	1,395.	2,250.	3,750.	1,079.	171,900.
25	15,000.	1,395.	2,250.	3,750.	749.	171,900.

Assumes all employees meet eligibility requirements, i.e., over 1,000 hours/year, minimum age and service requirements. Plans can be combined to maximize your goals.
Defined Benefit and Tandem Plans are not integrated, which is usually advisable.
If your income is consistent and you want to fund a lot towards retirement and have young employees or a few employees and are over age 45 to 50, check out a Defined Benefit or Target Benefit Plan.
Defined Benefit Plan assumes earnings of 7%.
From Pension Service Design, Inc., Suttons Bay, MI. With permission.

A retirement plan consultant will help you draw up the summary plan description, which must be given to employees describing the specifics of your plan. Also, your employees must receive an annual statement of values of the retirement plan. In addition, certain forms must be filed with the IRS, DOL, and/or Pension Benefit Guaranty Corporation to ensure proper qualification of your tax deductible contributions.

You must have a trust and a trustee or trustees for your retirement plan. You can hire a bank's trust department, independent trust company, name someone else as your trustee, be your own trustee, or a combination of the above, depending on your specific needs and wants. In our office we generally have the client be the trustee and then use an independent trust company or custodian company to do the accounting on the plans. We have worked out a relationship with a large trust company to do our trust accounting for our clients for a modest annual fee. This frees them to choose specific investment managers and frees us from the burden of doing the accounting on the plan, since this is all supplied by the trust company. This trust accounting service by banks is often called self-directed trusts. This allows you to have the flexibility of hiring one or a number of money managers and allows you to purchase passive investments or active investments in your portfolio and to diversify to your heart's content, without having to hassle with the tremendous bookkeeping expenses of having a number of investments. If your trust company will do it for $45 a year it's a bargain, and because you will be more likely to diversify and invest properly, it should also help increase your total portfolio returns.

The annual fee to have your plan administered should be around $300-$500, depending upon your number of employees and the complexity of the plan. If it's a defined benefit plan, the cost can go up to $1,500-$2,000 a year, depending on the complexity of your defined benefit plan. Shop around for plan services, but keep in mind the cost of having a plan administered should not be the determinant in choosing a retirement plan consulting firm.

Understand that usually banks, insurance companies, brokerage firms, etc., will have a lower fee schedule since their goal is to attract your money so that they can earn the investment fees and/or commissions on your funds. There are many fine independent companies that can provide services. In addition, there are many companies that do provide investment services that have a very favorable fee structure for administering your plan, in addition to doing a very fine job of advising you on your plan's investments.

If you are going to receive investment advice from the company that is providing your retirement plan services, make sure that they are registered investment advisors and are a competent firm.

WHICH PLAN IS THE BEST FOR YOU?

The plan that is best for you will depend on your specific circumstances; however, it is important to understand the three basic types of retirement plans.

Profit Sharing Plans

The profit sharing plan's key characteristic is that contributions are not fixed, and thus, can vary from year to year. The maximum that you can put in is 15 percent of total compensation of all employees covered under the plan. Profit sharing plans are especially good for younger physicians and physicians who want maximum flexibility.

Money Purchase Plans

Money purchase plans are similar to profit sharing plans; however, a money purchase plan is a fixed obligation. Money purchase contributions can be as high as 25 percent of total covered compensation. This allows an additional 10 percent to go into a retirement plan over a profit sharing plan. The maximum contribution to either a profit sharing plan or money purchase plan is $30,000 and often you will see a person with a fixed-obligation money purchase plan at 10 percent that is integrated with social security in tandem with a profit sharing plan that has the flexibility of going up to 15 percent in additional contributions. Thus, you have a fixed obligation on an annual basis of approximately 10 percent, while you can go up to 25 percent if you desire. This makes it very easy to plan and also makes it so that there will be less anxiety about having to contribute a substantial amount of money to the plan on an annual basis.

Defined Benefit Plan

The defined benefit plan benefits are based on the ultimate benefit that the plan will provide. For example, if your current salary is $90,000 a year, the defined benefit plan could be set up to provide you with up to a $90,000 annual benefit. Thus, the pension plan consultant would hire an actuary to determine the specific amount of money that must be set aside annually to make sure that you will have enough money in the trust to provide you with $90,000 annual income, or whatever amount you choose. These plans generally benefit older employees, or physicians, who are over the age of 50. Defined benefit plans can be very expensive to administer; however, they are very efficient wealth accumulators and work fantastically under certain circumstances. A good retirement plan consultant will run the numbers on a defined benefit plan if he or she feels that it is something that should be considered. Make sure that you understand that your fees will be roughly $1,000 greater than they would be under a money purchase or profit sharing plan.

Table 17-5 illustrates the different types of retirement plans and the specific amounts that can be contributed to the different plans, based on salaries and ages. This should help you get a greater understanding of the specific contribution limitations on these retirement plans.

There are many fine books out on pension planning and one of them is *Successful Pension Design For The Small to Medium-Sized Company* (Englewood Cliffs, NJ: Simmons Institute for Business Planning, IBP Plaza). These books should help you understand retirement and the specifics of retirement plans better. Because laws and nuances that affect retirement plans are ever-changing, it is best to hire a good, competent retirement plan consulting firm to assist you in your plan design and administration.

RETIREMENT PLANNING—THE LAST FIVE
(AND MOST IMPORTANT) YEARS

Dr. Jenkins was 55-years-old; his children were out of college; his mortgage payments were modest. With little short-term debt, he could easily live on the $100,000 annual income he was paying himself out of his PC. One day he lamented, "I probably should just retire now, since I only need $50,000 a year to live on. And, of the extra I earn, I pay $20,000 of it in taxes."

The doctor explained that he was going to take early retirement from his profit sharing and pension plan and retire in five years at the age of sixty. He was frustrated because, although he wanted to lower his salary, lowering it would also lower the amount he put into his retirement plan, and leave his retirement income inadequate for retiring at age sixty. He felt he was between a rock and a hard place.

For Dr. Jenkins, changing his retirement plan to a defined benefit plan would be ideal. On his current $100,000 income he was putting $25,000 into his pension and profit sharing plan. Under a defined benefit plan, the doctor could lower his salary to $55,000 and shelter $70,000 annually, which would provide him with a significantly greater retirement benefit at age 60 than his old plan.

In addition to the new defined benefit plan, his old pension and profit sharing plan's assets would keep growing over that 5 year period. If they earned a 12 percent return, the $200,000 in the trust could grow to about $380,000, providing him with $3,000-$4,000 additional monthly income.

Combining the income provided from all of his retirement plans, Dr. Jenkins, at age 60, could reasonably expect a retirement income in excess of $7,000 a month. At Social Security's eligibility age, his income would be further increased. Under the old retirement plan, the doctor would have been able to retire with about $4,000 monthly at age 60. Also, he was paying $20,000 annually in unnecessary taxes. Under the tax deferral benefit of his new retirement plan, Dr. Jenkins was able to defer that income into his retirement years, thus being able to spend that $7,000 a month sailing the out islands of the Caribbean.

IRA FACTS

An IRA Was Easy to Understand—After TRA/86
It's a Bit More Tricky

An IRA is a trust or custodial account you establish for yourself (and a beneficiary, if you wish). You make cash contributions into the IRA and direct the trustee to purchase one or more investments for the account. Your investments remain in the account until you withdraw them (usually when you retire).

The rules governing IRAs are numerous. Once you understand them, however, you can make your IRA the ultimate retirement planning tool. Here is a brief rundown.

Limits on Deductibility

IRAs for years prior to 1987 are 100 percent tax deductible up to a $2,000 contribution limit or 100 percent of earned income if less than $2,000 and $2,250 for an employee and a nonworking spouse. Tax Reform Act 1986 has complicated IRAs for years after 1986. If your joint adjusted gross income is less than $40,000, you can deduct 100 percent of your IRA up to $2,000 regardless of whether you or your spouse are covered under a pension plan. If your joint income is over $40,000, but less than $50,000, your IRA deductions are scaled down proportionately (i.e., income of $45,000) then half of your IRA is deductible. If you and your spouse earn $50,000 or more adjusted gross income, and one of you is covered under a company sponsored pension plan, regardless of which spouse earns what part of the income, both you and your spouse will be ineligible to deduct your IRA.

If you and/or your spouse are not covered under a company retirement plan you can deduct your IRA as you would prior to 1987. Up to $2,000 each or 100 percent of income, maximum $2,000 per IRA or $2,250 if you have a nonworking spouse could be deducted.

Single nonmarried tax payers can deduct their IRA as before 1987 if they earn less than $25,000 and even if they are covered under a pension plan. If a single person earns between $25,000 and $30,000, his or her deduction will be proportionate as with a joint filer. If you are not covered under a retirement plan you can still deduct up to $2,000 or 100 percent of your income, whichever is less. Regardless of your income or if you are covered under a plan and your earnings are over $30,000, you can still get that tax-free growth on your IRA although you don't get the current deduction.

Funding

You may contribute a maximum of $2,000 or 100 percent of your compensation or alimony, whichever is less, to your IRA each year. No matter how many IRAs you have, your contribution can't exceed the annual ceiling.

If your spouse does not work, you can contribute to a "spousal" IRA for him or her. Your total annual contributions to both your accounts may not exceed $2,250, and no more than $2,000 can go into either account. If you are both employed, you each may put $2,000 a year, or 100 percent of your income (if less) into your separate IRAs.

Eligibility

Anyone under age 70 ½ who earns compensation (wages, salary, tips, commissions, and other "earned income") or collects alimony can set up an IRA.

Trustees

You may not hold or invest your IRA money yourself. The law requires that you place it in the hands of a qualified trustee or custodian—a bank (including savings institutions and credit unions), trust company, insurance company, brokerage firm, or other financial organizations that meet IRA requirements.

Deposit Deadline

You can establish and contribute to an IRA anytime during the year or up until April 15 of the following year and still claim the deduction for the year.

Withdrawals and Penalties

If you withdraw money before you are age 59 ½ or permanently disabled, you will pay a 10 percent penalty tax in addition to the ordinary income tax on the amount withdrawn. From age 59 ½ to 70 ½, you can withdraw as much or as little as you like at any time. (At no time, however, may you borrow money from your IRA or pledge it as collateral for a loan.)

Once you pass age 70 ½, you are required to withdraw at least a minimum amount each year, based on an IRS table of average life expectancies. Each year you can calculate the amount to be withdrawn.

Under the Tax Reform Act of 1986, (1) all IRAs are treated as one contract; (2) all distributions during a taxable year are treated as one distribution, and (3) amounts paid from an IRA are included in gross income and taxed under annuity rules. Table 17-6 is an example.

Seven Myths About IRAS

The entire subject of individual retirement accounts is a source of confusion and apprehension for many investors. The advertising blitz staged by many financial institutions to attract IRA deposits has done little to dispel popular misconceptions. The Tax Reform Act of 1986 has also made IRAs more confusing than ever. Here are a few of the most common fallacies about IRAs:

Table 17-6

	Tax Deductible Contributions	Tax Free Growth	Non-Deductible Contributions	Withdrawals	End of Year Account Value
1. 1987 Dr. Jones makes a $2,000 IRA deposit—$1,500 is deductible, $500 is not	+ $1,500		+ $500		$2,000
2. It grows to + $2,200 by the end of 1987		+ $200			2,200
3. 1988 Dr. Jones makes a $2,000 non-deductible contribution			+ 2,000		
4. IRA grows to $4,600 by end of 1988		+ 400			4,600
5. 1989 Dr. Jones draws out $1,000 from his IRA				- $1,000	
6. By the end of 1989 his IRA grows to $4,000 even after his $1,000 withdrawal		+ 400			4,000
TOTALS	1,5000	$1,000	2,500	1,000	4,000
		$2,500		$5,000	
		$2,500 ÷ $5,000 = 50%			

You take the tax free growth and deductible contribution and divide them by your total withdrawals + plan value at the end of the year to get the amount of your IRA that is deductible. Thus, if half of your IRA was made up of non-deductible contributions and the balance was deductible contributions and earnings when you cashed your plan in, half would be taxable and the other half not.

Note: There are many laws affecting IRAs and this chart does not cover all of them. Seek professional help when setting up your IRA.

From Pension Service Design, Inc., Suttons Bay, MI. With permission.

1. *An IRA is a lot of trouble to start and keep.* An IRA is actually one of the easiest ways to invest your money. The trustee of your account does most of the work for you.
2. *IRAs are only for oldtimers approaching retirement.* You will forfeit the greatest benefits of tax-free compounding of earnings if you put off starting your IRA. The sooner you start making contributions, the bigger you account will grow . . . and that first deposit can make a dramatic difference.
3. *I am already covered by a Pension and Profit Sharing Retirement Plan and my wife and I earn over $50,000 so my IRA will not be deductible. However, because of the tax deferred growth on IRA contributions for 1987 and beyond, we*

still plan on funding our IRAs. Non-deductible IRA contributions are not a good idea since TRA/86 had a few tax "whammies" that could substantially negate the benefits at retirement of the tax-free compounding on non-deductible IRAs. A better bet for non-deductible contributions would be a tax deferred annuity that gives tax free growth and does not have any contribution limit.

4. *An IRA locks up your money until you retire.* While a tax penalty discourages using an IRA for short-term investing, you may withdraw money from your account any time you need to. By keeping your money in an IRA, you can beat the return on an ordinary taxable investment in less time than you think.

5. *IRAs do not generate high investment yields.* If your investment horizons do not extend beyond your corner bank's certificate of deposit, you're right. Treat your IRA as seriously as any other major investment. If your account isn't earning as much as it should, do something about it.

6. *An IRA restricts investment flexibility.* Quite to the contrary, an IRA is one of the most versatile tax-deferred retirement plans available because you can control the investments.

7. *You should delay contributing to your IRA as long as possible.* If you put off funding your IRA, you'll lose money. The sooner you contribute, the more you'll have later on.

18

Who Should Manage Your Retirement Plan?

The person (or persons) you choose to make the day-to-day investment decisions regarding your retirement plan portfolio represents the single most important factor affecting your investment portfolio's performance. As Aldous Huxley said, "There is no substitute for talent." In today's volatile investment market, it can be very expensive to make the wrong choices. The fact is, most investment managers are not selected properly.

Preserving the purchasing power of your investment dollars is no easy task. Sooner or later you and your employees will be receiving benefits from your retirement plan trust. If your trust investments have not been managed effectively, you could end up facing very costly consequences and, perhaps, some unhappy employees.

The Employees Retirement Income Security Act (ERISA) of 1974 requires careful and prudent administration exclusively for the benefit of plan participants and holds you, as the plan sponsor, liable for that administration. ERISA makes the plan sponsor liable for that administration. ERISA makes plan sponsors fiduciaries and binds them to follow the prudent man rule.

For 150 years fiduciaries have been guided by the prudent man rule laid down by Judge Samuel Putnam of the Massachusetts Supreme Judicial Court in 1831. He stated:

> All that can be required of a trustee to invest is that he shall conduct himself faithfully and exercise a sound discretion. He is to observe how men of prudence, discretion and intelligence manage their own affairs, not in regard to speculation, but in regard to the permanent disposition of their funds considering the probable income as well as the probable safety, of the capital to be invested.

When the prudent man rule was originally written, retirement plan funds as we know them today, did not exist. The rule was designed for other types of fiduciaries such as trustees of charities and educational funds and estates of widows and orphans.

ERISA in 1974 added requirements that specifically apply to retirement plans. These guidelines are:

1. A fiduciary shall discharge his duties with respect to a plan solely in the interest of the participants and the beneficiaries for the exclusive purpose of:
    a. providing benefits to participants and their beneficiaries, and,
    b. defraying reasonable expenses of administering the plan. . .
2. . . . with the care, skill, prudence and diligence under the circumstances then prevailing that a prudent man, acting in a like capacity and familiar with such matters, would use in the conduct of an enterprise of a like character and with like aims. . .
3. . . . by diversifying the investments of the plan so as to minimize the risk of large losses unless under the circumstances it is clearly prudent not to do so. Section 404(a)(1) of ERISA.

As a result of this section of ERISA:

1. The fiduciary must take special care not to favor specific firms or individuals because of bias or friendship.
2. Give undue weighting to established credit or bank relationships, either company or personal.
3. Make choices motivated by self-interest or other extraneous considerations. For example, it may seem to make good sense for you to have your pension plan assets managed by the same bank that handles your payroll, provides you with a line of credit and perhaps, the mortgage on your home. Under ERISA, your existing relationship with the bank is not a proper consideration in deciding who will be entrusted with the management of your retirement plan assets.

Simply stated, ERISA requires that a retirement plan fiduciary should identify the retirement plan's investment objectives and guide its investment program accordingly. The fiduciary should effectively monitor and supervise the ongoing investment programs and consider the needs of participants and beneficiaries. The fiduciary should make sure the funds are properly diversified and has sound portfolio balance between common stocks, bonds, money market instruments, etc.

A fiduciary should not invest too large a portion of the plan's assets in the security of any one company or industry and the fiduciary should make sure the assets are suitably allocated among various types of investments, to hold down risks while providing the much needed, adequate diversification.

In addition, if you are a plan fiduciary, you should keep documented records of how and why the plan's investment program was selected and how it is being monitored.

What is an acceptable rate of return for a retirement plan fund? As a general yardstick for measuring performance, you should: (1) strive to have a total return that exceeds the average annual rate of return on 90-day Treasury bonds, which are completely risk-free investments over a five year or longer period, and (2) have a representative rate of return on top of inflation of perhaps 3-6 percent over this period.

The investment markets are not managed, your portfolio is, and you should expect to have above-average performance. Investment managers cannot control inflation, volatile interest rates, or the many economic, political or social forces that affect the investment markets every day. They can stay abreast of significant forces and events and with foresight, experience, talent, time and flexibility, they can make wise and timely investment decisions to maximize the potential for investment gains.

Choosing the right advisor for your retirement plan can be a hassle. There are basically six different choices which you can make:

1. Manage the money yourself or hire a:
2. Bank trust company
3. Brokerage firm subsidiary
4. Independent advisory firm
5. Mutual fund
6. Insurance company

First, you can manage the money yourself. Unless you and one of your PC colleagues are the only beneficiaries of the trust, however, you must strictly adhere to your fiduciary responsibilities to choose what's best for the beneficiaries of the trust. If you feel you are the best person to manage the funds then you must be able to justify your stand.

BANK TRUST COMPANY

Bank trust departments are probably the first choice of most individuals for money management help. Usually the bank trust companies are chosen as an investment manager not because of their performance, but rather for convenience. Unfortunately, most banks' investment performance has been comparatively poor. Perhaps banks' poor performance comes because banks are in the business of lending money and providing other financial services. The trust department is a service provided that often is not a substantial profit center and does not get the attention the other departments of the bank get.

Many larger banks manage too much money to perform well and instead of choosing clients selectively and providing individualized management, banks tend to accept all accounts and treat them alike, often directing new money to their comingled funds, which are somewhat similar to mutual funds. Usually the talent of the bank is spread too thin to provide any personal attention and the investment policies are often too bureaucratic and cumbersome to make rapid portfolio changes on a day-to-day basis. Decision making in the bank is often hampered by committees that are unwieldy with a deep rooted fear of litigation. Usually it is very hard to find consistent, predictable management in banks and in most cases, you should use your bank for its strength in lending and checking but let other investment specialists manage your funds. By looking beyond your bank you probably can increase the likelihood of satisfactory yields. Naturally there are exceptions to this rule and some banks, especially in recent years, have strived to upgrade their investment performance by hiring some top money managers and.giving them tremendous freedom over client accounts. Your new bank trust department may change its facade, but make sure under its facade, there really were legitimate changes made.

BROKERAGE FIRM SUBSIDIARIES

Many securities' dealers have established investment advisory subsidiaries. Brokerage firm subsidiaries have access to tremendous amounts of information about investments and there are a wide variety of services the money managers in brokerage firm subsidiaries provide. Some brokerage firm management subsidiaries allow portfolio supervisors tremendous autonomy and are run similarly to the small, independent money management firms. Often the brokerage firm's money managers come from private investment counseling firms that had superior results and were aggressively recruited by the brokerage firm for prestige, etc.

One major drawback of subsidiaries of brokerage firms is the advisors' limited access to independent analytical data. Independent investment advisors often purchase outside research with commission dollars and sometimes, broker affiliates channel their commission dollars to their parent firm so the money to purchase this independent research is often scarce. Naturally, some firms purchase all their stocks through firms other than their parent to overcome this concern of their clients. Analyze a brokerage manager as you would the independent manager or mutual fund.

INDEPENDENT INVESTMENT ADVISORS

Just as with brokerage firms or bank trust departments, with independent advisors it is important to check out the people that will be managing your money, and not just the firm. In the investment management business, whether you hire a brokerage firm, bank or independent firm, biggest is not the same as best. Any large investment management firm that manages huge amounts of money often faces the same problems that large bank trust departments do, i.e., limited liquidity, excess workloads, and, sometimes, a less experienced staff.

Firms managing the very high dollar volume of assets are often limited in their choices regarding their portfolio weighting towards smaller company stocks because by buying and selling huge amounts of one company's security, they could have an effect upon the price swings of that security.

According to Bob Jeavons, a portfolio manager for Alpine Capital Management Corporation in Colorado, a general rule among portfolio managers is to avoid investment positions in excess of 2 days trading volume or 10 percent of the outstanding shares, which for firms with huge amounts of money under management, could cause them to compromise their investment strategy towards larger capitalized investments in order to manage funds responsibly. Their size limits their ability to act quickly in response to market changes, i.e., the buying or selling of huge amounts of stock can affect the market in such a way as to have a negative result on investment performance. Size measured by either assets managed or clients serviced can often be a handicap more than an advantage. Large firms are more likely to treat you as a problem rather than an opportunity since you're just one of a large number of clients. Usually the larger firms have minimum investment accounts of between $250,000 and $1,000,000 under management, which makes their minimum account size prohibitive for smaller plans.

If you are choosing an investment management firm, don't consider only the most well-known firms, because then you're buying the firm's name rather than performance. Some well-known firms have mediocre track records and great marketing programs. Don't consider a firm just because it's in your local area. Of the hundreds of investment advisory firms in the US, most offer mediocre or average performance. You should not let civic pride or the emotional comfort of physical proximity limit your opportunity for superior results. When you look at the mechanics of the investment advisory relationship, geographical proximity becomes insignificant. Assets usually are held by a custodial bank. Your securities' transactions are handled by brokerage firms and usually, your advisory firm has limited power of attorney so it can't authorize payments of cash or securities to any third party for any other reason than a security transaction. The security is always registered in the name of your trust and no matter where your advisory firm is located, it is just a phone call away. Most communication is by phone or mail anyway and your advisor can meet with you regularly when they visit your area of the country.

Don't choose the money management firm based on past performance alone. Determine whether their past performance was done by the person or persons that will be managing your money. Also, if the firm has grown significantly in recent years, be sure to ask the manager how they have handled this growth and why they feel the performance of the future can be as great as the past, now that they have more money under management, which could hamper their ability to get in or out of the common stock and bond markets quickly.

Don't consider only older, established firms. Usually we tend to associate longevity with stability. But in investment advisory firms, money management is an entrepreneural task and there is no evidence that portfolio management can be institutionalized with success. Firms don't produce superior investment results, individual advisors do. If a firm has been in existence for 50 years, how many of the original principals do you suppose are still actively managing the portfolios? It's likely that the only continuity that now exists is the firm's name.

If deciding to change managers, don't procrastinate—it's very easy to fall into that trap. Often a physician will rationalize putting off an investment advisory decision for another year and inertia can have disastrous consequences. For example, some of the excuses for waiting are:

- "Interest rates are high now so there's no reasons to change."
- "There's another new trust officer at the bank and he or she needs some smart-up time."
- "Our committee won't meet until next fall."
- "Our present advisors have done poorly so far, but in fairness we'll give them some more time. Maybe they'll do better next year."
- "Our bank's trust departments performance has been poor but the bank is our first line of credit."
- "I'm on the board of directors at the bank that manages our money so there's no chance we can change investment advisors now."
- "The market is too low to change now."
- "The market is too high to change now."
- "The market is stagnant so I shouldn't change now."
- "No one else can do any better for us."
- "Making a change will take too much time and be a hassle."
- "We're too busy now to discuss our employee benefit fund."
- "We'll defer this to a later meeting."
- "I think I'll go play racquetball."

MUTUAL FUNDS

Huge amounts of retirement plan monies have been invested in mutual funds, often because retirement plan fiduciaries are dissatisfied with the investment performance of their money managers, either through banks or independents. There are hundreds of mutual funds, many of which specialize in investing retirement plan monies.

Mutual funds are often categorized by risk. You as a fiduciary can compare mutual funds based on the portfolio risk you desire as learned earlier. A mutual fund designation of aggressive or maximum capital gains should not be compared to a mutual fund with a designation of income/-bond specialization since the maximum capital gains fund, which takes on more risk, will logically have better investment performance over an extended period of time than a fund that was invested with substantially less risk, i.e., a bond fund. It's not fair to compare an investment that has substantial risk to a fund with very little risk such as a money market fund. Mutual funds taken as a group have generally outperformed both bank pooled funds and insurance company funds. This performance is not hard to understand. The mutual fund industry has tremendous assets under management. Some have many billions of dollars all managed with a low average annual management fee of ½ percent to 1 ½ percent of assets under management. These firms have millions of dollars with which to hire the very finest "cream of the crop" from the investment professional pool.

Mutual funds however, can suffer from the same problems bank trust companies and the large independent money managers can suffer from—success. Often after a mutual fund becomes very large, it has trouble being nimble and quick, i.e., getting in or out of the market or buying the stocks in smaller companies. Often in choosing mutual funds, it's best to choose a mutual fund with the smaller asset size so that your manager can get in and out of the different investments without having an effect on the markets.

When analyzing a mutual fund, you're buying a specific manager or group of managers, thus you should assure yourself just as you would with an independent money manager, that the manager that gave the mutual fund its spectacular performance is still managing that fund. If you find that the manager has moved to another fund then you should invest in the new fund since its asset base would be small and the old fund would be getting a new, perhaps marginal, money manager.

Mutual funds offer quite a number of conveniences. You can look in almost any newspaper on a business day and find out the value of your fund. Many mutual funds let you change your mind and move your money among their other specialized funds such as growth mutual fund shares, international stocks and bond funds, income common stock funds, U.S. government bond funds, etc., with a phone call.

In fact, some investment management firms have their clients stick their money into a mutual fund group with a number of different specialized funds and then the money manager allocates their money between the funds as they feel the market warrants. Most mutual funds let you move your money among their funds at no charge or a modest $5 charge per move, which is much less expensive than the commission charge if you were to move large blocks of common stocks.

INSURANCE COMPANIES

The last type of investment choice is insurance companies. Many insurance companies also manage mutual funds in addition to portfolio management subsidiaries and they should be analyzed as described earlier in this article. Insurance companies historically have not had performance as favorable as the mutual funds. However, insurance companies do offer some specialized services that are not accessible at a bank or through a mutual fund.

Insurance companies offer investment contracts that guarantee you a minimum rate of return. These investment contracts can range from a 6 month guaranteed rate of return to a longer term guaranteed rate of return, with a fluctuating return that could allow your investment return to be greater than the minimum guarantees.

When buying any insurance company product, you should first make sure the company is financially sound and then you should check the company's fees. Insurance companies often have substantial fees for getting in and out of their investments. Often these fees can range from 5-30 percent of the value of your investment fund, so ask your insurance advisors about those costs before making any investment in insurance company products.

Finding an investment manager can be a time-consuming endeavor. Some investment firms specialize in keeping a list of investment advisory firms whom they've checked out for their clients. Often if you call a pension consulting firm, they can give you a list of referrals, or ask your broker, financial planner, or a colleague.

There are also a few specialized firms in the country that keep a stable of money managers whom they analyze on a continual basis, and, for a fee, they will supply you with the statistical data on these fund managers. After you have received the names of some money managers, check them out carefully.

Never hire a manager based on fees alone. Expect to pay for what you get. If your old manager charges ½ percent on the amount under management annually and the firm you are considering charges 2 percent, or four times as much, don't throw them out automatically. If you feel that the new company's performance will be greater by a few percents than your old company, then you got a deal. Fees are deductible so if your charges go up a bit, remember the government will pay a large proportion of the expense.

Once you hire your manager, if you have a concern or don't understand a transaction they make, call your manager and have him or her explain what and why they did what they did. You should expect to have your phone calls answered promptly by your manager and all problems attended to in a timely manner. There will be problems such as late or improper statements, improperly made transactions, and so on. You shouldn't expect these problems not to happen, but you should expect them to be resolved in a timely manner.

You should understand the transactions that are made in your account. If you don't, have your manager explain all transactions you do not understand. If you have little understanding of investment markets, have your manager suggest a few books you can read to increase your understanding.

Money management is more art than science and your manager will make lots of mistakes. That is part of the game. Even the best managers will buy some investments at $20 and sell at $12. Expect it.

Watch your portfolio's overall performance. One of our clients, who has had a number of managers invest his PC's retirement funds over the years, puts it, "If you watch each investment in your portfolio daily, you'll soon put yourself on Inderal."

Retirement plans are invested for long-term results, so don't be too worried about the day-to-day fluctuations in the markets; that's your manager's job. He or she is being paid to consternate over your portfolio. Another client puts it this way: "I feel secure knowing that my money manager is losing sleep when the financial markets are in disarray. Isn't that what I pay him for . . . so I can sleep?"

19

Estate Planning (spend it now, the kids don't need it

Everyone who acquires assets is involved in estate planning. The form in which you own or take title to those assets is a part of an estate plan. Everyone has an estate plan either by design or default. In approaching an intentional estate plan there are four general questions to answer.

1. What is your estate and who owns it?
2. What are your objectives?
3. What is your present estate plan?
4. Which of the available tools will best accomplish your objectives?

A typical estate consists of some or all of the following assets: home, other real estate, furnishings and personal property, vehicles and recreational equipment, cash, checking and savings accounts, stocks and bonds, insurance, retirement plans, mortgages, notes, land contracts, oil interests. All of these assets that are owned by you comprise your estate. If some or all of these assets are owned jointly with another person they are still part of your estate for some purposes (i.e., for tax purposes but not for probate purposes) and the form of ownership determines what happens to those assets in the event of your death. The first step in preparing to do your estate planning is to make a list of your assets with values. This can be done on an asset schedule such as the one in Figure 19-1. This will serve as a starting point for an estate planning discussion with your advisors and will also constitute a permanent inventory of your estate that can be updated from time to time as it changes and reviewed for the need for any new planning.

After you have determined what your estate consists of you must decide what are your objectives in your estate plan. Four general and common objectives are as follows:

1. Creating and conserving the estate for the benefit of your family. Reviewing what you own and how.
2. Provide orderly disposition of those assets to whom you wish them to go.

Property, listing in order: real estate, household furnishings, autos, jewelry, valuable collections, bank accounts, bonds, stocks, business interests, and any other property:

EXAMPLE

Item	Current Market Value	Original Cost	Location	Ownership
Home	$30,000	$20,000	15 N. 5th St.	Husband and wife
Busines	35,000	5,000	203 Main Street	Husband
H/hold furniture	2,000	4,000	At home	Husband and wife
Checking account	500	500	1st National Bank	Husband and wife
Stamp collection	600	500	At home	Wife
Savings account	1,200	1,200	Citizens Bank	Husband
Seried "E" Bonds	1,500	1,200	Safety Deposit Box	Husband
AT&T stock	3,500	1,500	Safety Deposit Box	Wife and son

For completion by you as in example above.

Item	Current Market Value	Original Cost	Location	Ownership

Estimated Debts and Mortgages against your Estate.

(Excluding ordinary household expenses.)

Debt or Mortgage to: Present Balance

_____ $ _____

_____ $ _____

_____ $ _____

Fig. 19-1. Asset ownership chart.

3. Reducing taxes and costs to a minimum.
4. Providing for management of estate by a competent personal representative/trustee for the benefit of your beneficiaries.

You may obviously have other more specific or more important objectives considering the type of estate, size of estate, and specific needs or desires of your family. It is important to review with your advisors in detail your objectives so that the estate plan that is prepared for you meets those objectives and is not a form of standard estate plan designed without the benefit of this discussion.

Figures 19-2 through 19-5 illustrate specific estates and sample simplified estate plans used to help each client achieve his or her goals. These sample estate plans should be used as an educational tool by you to get a feel for how specific planning strategies can help you. After you have determined what your objectives are and have reviewed your estate with your advisor, you should determine what your present estate plan is. This may consist of a Will and/or Trust that may need to be updated. Your estate plan may simply consist of the form of ownership in which you hold your assets. For instance, the law of your state may provide that assets that you hold as joint tenant with full rights of survivorship upon your death will pass automatically to that other joint owner. If you hold title to real estate, for instance, as tenants in common rather than as joint tenants with full right of survivorship then your interest in that asset will be a part of your estate rather than passing to the other co-owner. These and other rules of the law depend upon state law and need to be reviewed in detail with your advisors to determine what your present estate plan is.

Another example of your present estate plan that may have been created without intentional planning is the beneficiary designations on your life insurance. You should obviously review with your advisors your life insurance to determine whether you have enough or too much coverage and to determine whether you have designated the proper beneficiaries to accomplish your wishes. The designation of beneficiaries can obviously have estate planning consequences and tax consequences as well.

If you have had a will prepared, or other estate planning documents, you should review with your advisors your present estate structure and objectives and changes in the law since the date of those documents to determine whether or not any changes are necessary. It is also important to review any changes in your estate or family situation that may require changes in your present plan. If you do not have a Will or Trust, or other estate planning documents that have been prepared for you, you nevertheless have an estate plan that can be referred to as the state plan. State law determines for people who die intestate, that is without a Will, who will receive those assets owned by the deseased. Since this law is inflexible and is written to apply to general situations and does not take into consideration any special circumstances involving your estate and/or

Dr. Capron, age 35—Kim (Spouse), age 34
Child, age 1—One is on the way

$ 2,000. IRA
$ 150,000. Home & Personal
$ 100,000. Debts
$ 250,000. Insurance

GOALS
1. Income to spouse @ $ 5,000.
2. Monthly debts paid.
3. Educate children.
4. Save estate and death costs.

- Wills naming guardians for children, designating debts be paid and assets to pass to surviving spouse and/or children.
- Name Kim as beneficiary of IRA
- Raise Insurance Death Benefit to $ 1,150,000.

Dr. Capron's Death

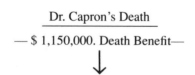

— $ 1,150,000. Death Benefit—

$ 150,000. to spouse outright to pay debts
and provide some liquidity

$ 400,000. income to spouse.

$ 600,000 to Dr. Capron's family trust to
benefit Dr. Capron's spouse and children.

Income to family for health, maintenance,
educations, and support at
approximately $ 5,000./mo.

Fig. 19-2.

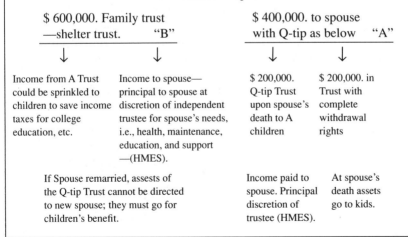

Dr. Lindee, age 40—Spouse, age 35
3 Children, ages 5, 7, and 10

$ 50,000. IRA & Pension
$ 100,000. Home & Personal—Net (Joint)
$ 1,000,000. Insurance to revocable trust
as illustrated below

Number one goal is financial security and income to spouse and kids.

Strategies to consider:

• Porover will with guardians named.
• IRA and Pension's primary beneficiary is spouse, secondary is Trust

NOTE: regarding estate taxes, first
death—estate tax is "$0." Second death
approximately $ 50,000.

NOTE: Spouse's income at 6% = $ 60,000.
Trust can limit income if desired, i.e.,
.005% of trust corpus paid monthly, etc.

— $ 1,000,000.—
Paid to Revocable Living Trust
With A-B Split

$ 600,000. Family trust
—shelter trust.   "B"

$ 400,000. to spouse
with Q-tip as below   "A"

↓   ↓   ↓   ↓

Income from A Trust
could be sprinkled to
children to save income
taxes for college
education, etc.

Income to spouse—
principal to spouse at
discretion of independent
trustee for spouse's needs,
i.e., health, maintenance,
education, and support
—(HMES).

$ 200,000.
Q-tip Trust
upon spouse's
death to A
children

$ 200,000. in
Trust with
complete
withdrawal
rights

If Spouse remarried, assests of
the Q-tip Trust cannot be directed
to new spouse; they must go for
children's benefit.

Income paid to
spouse. Principal
discretion of
trustee (HMES).

At spouse's
death assets
go to kids.

Fig. 19-3.

Dr. Smith, age 55—Jean (Spouse), age 53
5 Children, all grown and on their own

$ 1,000,000. IRAs & Pension
$ 350,000. Net Equity of personal and
home owned JT. Wros.
$ 750,000. Investments owned personally
(mostly JT. Wros.)
$ 150,000. Group insurance on Dr. Smith to Age 65

GOALS

1. Lifetime income to spouse of $ 90,000. annually.
2. Help grandchildren with college.
3. Benefit charity with part of money, now and in future.
4. Balance of estate to children
5. Save estate and gift taxes.
6. Want to keep working until age 65 and want income at age 65 to be $90,000. in today's money.
7. Reduce personal taxes now.

STRATEGIES TO CONSIDER (oversimplified):

At Dr. Smith's death:

- $ 1,000,000. in retirement plan assets to Jean—10 year average and/or roll over to IRA—Draw on assets as needed. This asset will help provide $ 90,000. annual income—Jean named beneficiary of these assets.
- $ 350,000. in home and personal assets would go to Jean outright through joint ownership. Thes assets would go to children by will.
- $ 750,000. Investments—sever Jt. Tenants and go with Tenants in Common. Half to Dr. Smith and half to Jean distributed as below.

Dr. Smith: Half @	$ 375,000.		Dr. Smith's grandchildren's
	charitable →	Income to →	educational crummy trust.
	trust		After youngest grandchild
			turns age 35, trust disposed
			to charity

On his death, remainder of trust to charity.

Jean: Half @ $375,000. transferred to living irrevocable trust.

Income to Jean and Dr. Smith during their lives and to children at death.
$ 150,000. insurance to living irrevocable trust.

Fig. 19-4.

Dr. John Leathers—Joanna Graham Leathers (Spouse)

John—$ 1,200,000. in assets
4 children (previous marriage) ages 18-24

Joanna—$ 100,000. in assets
2 children (previous marriage)

JOHN'S GOAL:
John wishes to provide for Joanna's security. If he dies first, he wants his assets to go to his children.

JOANNA'S GOAL:
Joanna wishes to have her assets all go to her children at her death equally.

JOHN'S PLAN:
—$ 1,200,000.—
—Revocable Living Trust—

$ 600,000. Q-tip	John's Death	$ 600,000 income to
income to wife.		children of John. None
No principal		to wife. Principal to
invasion		children at John's discretion.
"A" Trust		(Children's Trust)
		"B" Trust

Upon Joanna's Death
money to children's trust
(this would pay any estate
taxes).

JOANNA'S PLAN:
Joanna should have will leaving the $100,000 outright to her 2 children equally at her death.

John and Joanna sign a post nuptial agreement waiving their rights under state law to take part of the other's estate as a surviving spouse.

Fig. 19-5.

family situation it is important to understand the application of that state law in proceeding to design your estate plan.

Once you have determined what your estate consists of and what your estate planning objectives are and the laws applicable to your estate without planning, you can then review with your advisors the available estate planning tools that might best accomplish your wishes. Naturally you should prepare your family for your death and if you follow the guidelines of Figure 19-6, your family should be able to achieve financial normalcy after your death.

WILLS AND TRUSTS AND OTHER ESTATE PLANNING TOOLS

A Will is a document that you will sign and which will contain directions for the administration and disposition of your estate following your death by administration through Probate Court. A Will must be prepared according to the applicable state law. A Will does not enable a person to avoid probate but enables a person to set forth his wishes as to how his estate will be probated and to whom and when that estate will be distributed. Probate is the process that insures that the wishes expressed in the Will are carried out. By having a Will prepared for you and signing it, you are not restricted during your lifetime in terms of the ownership, administration, or disposition of any of the assets that you own or that may be covered in your Will. Your Will, although valid if prepared according to applicable state law, does not become effective until your death.

A Trust is a separate legal entity that you may create through the means of a trust document, either separately or as a part of your Will. The Trust may be in the form of a "testamentary" trust that is included as part of your Will and comes into existence following your death and after the probate of your estate. The Trust may also take the form of a living trust, also commonly referred to as a revocable living trust, which is a separate document from your Will and is funded during your lifetime. The revocable living trust is entirely revocable by you during your lifetime and to the extent that it is funded with your assets during your lifetime, all of those assets in the Trust will avoid probate at the time of your death since the Trust is a separate legal entity and its existence continues after your death. If you want to retain greater control over the Trust assets and administration beyond the revocability, you could name yourself as trustee and administer the trust assets during your lifetime with a successor trustee named in the document to automatically take over the administration of the trust assets immediately upon your death.

The Trust can also be used to accomplish estate tax planning objectives by dividing your estate following your death into separate shares for surviving spouse and children to reduce the tax incidence upon your death.

Estate Planning

1. Your spouse (father, mother, sibling, friend, children, etc.) should know whom to call if you die and where to look to find a list of your assets.
2. Your spouse should have a letter of instructions and whom you feel he/she should trust as an advisor for:

   a. accounting
   b. legal work
   c. investment advice
   d. insurance
   e. general finance planning help.

3. Also, he/she should know about funeral arrangements, i.e., cremation, burial, gifting of organs, cemetery, etc.
4. Your children should know whom you have named as guardians and with them you should discuss why you chose "Uncle Harvey and Aunt Mary."
5. You should have a "Letter of values" written to your guardians stating why you chose them to care for your children and discussing with them how you would like your children raised and your values, i.e., school, sports, college, private high schools, summer camp, driving, ability to visit relatives on other side of the family, etc.

Fig. 19-6. Estate planning.

The Trust, whether a living trust or a testamentary trust, may simply be designed for the purpose of receiving insurance proceeds following your death, and contain the directions for administration and distribution of those proceeds, with no other assets intended as trust funding. The Trust may be designed as an irrevocable trust, meaning a trust that cannot be revoked by you. An irrevocable trust may be appropriate if one of your objectives is to remove assets from your estate for the benefit of other beneficiaries without an immediate distribution outright to those beneficiaries. You may also accomplish estate reduction by means of outright gifts. If these gifts are less than $10,000 per donee they will not incur a gift tax. If the gifts are to charitable, religious, educational, or other such organizations, they may qualify for the income tax charitable deduction.

   Another important estate planning tool is a Durable Power of Attorney. This is a document wherein you designate someone else as your attorney-in-fact and give them limited or broad powers to handle your business affairs and perhaps make personal decisions for you in the event of your incompetency. Many state laws permit a Durable Power of Attorney. The Durable Power of Attorney is valid only during your lifetime and any authority granted in that document terminates upon your death. The use of a Durable Power of Attorney to protect during incompetency may also enable you to avoid the involvement of a probate court in the establishment of a guardianship or a conservatorship to supervise the administration of your estate or personal decisions during your period of incompetency. In addition to preparing legally for death, you should prepare your family emotionally.

20
Using Experts and Financial Planning Professionals

Once you have your written financial plan of action, your next step is to become a financial doer; and once you become a doer, it is important that you find competent professionals to assist you. The financial doing will be much easier if you have worked with a financial planner in drawing up your financial plan. However, regardless of whether you use a financial planner or not you will need to use outside experts in different fields to assist you in drawing your financial plan into action. For example, if you have decided that you need your wills revised and a trust drawn, you will need to hire a good, competent estate planning or tax attorney to assist you in drawing up the trust. If you decide that a retirement plan makes sense, you should hire a competent retirement planning consultant to assist you with the nuance of your plan.

Choosing professionals to assist you can be very trying; and a poorly qualified or domineering professional can raise havoc with even the best drawn financial plan. I remember asking an accountant why he hadn't recommended that his client incorporate in order to set up a more favorable retirement plan, saying "Paul, I know it would save my client a lot of money in taxes; however, if I saved him that money in taxes, he would just spend it on frivolous things." I then asked, "Isn't that his prerogative to spend his money as he wishes?" And he answered, "Paul, you don't understand, he would just waste that money, so what's the use of incorporating him or using tax saving strategies when he will just spend the money?" This accountant had been the advisor for this client for 30 years. This client came to me because he owed many years in back taxes.

By simply rearranging his financial situation, we were able to get his debt situation under control and make it so that he is accumulating wealth for retirement and also able to go off Inderol.

The accountant was very dominating, and when I confronted him in front of my client, regarding the remarks that he made, he denied each word.

Another incident involves an insurance agent who called himself a financial advisor; he recommended that a client of his buy a large whole life policy as a panacea to take care of his need for disability income, life insurance, retirement plan, and a need to build liquid cash.

The insurance agent had him pay for this insurance benefit on a non-deductible basis. When I asked the agent why he hadn't recommended that the client purchase term insurance, a real disability policy, and then put the rest of the money into a retirement plan, his reply was, "Paul, no one can make any money just selling term insurance and earning the small commissions on securities that would go into a retirement plan." Each of these advisors, if they could be called advisors, had known their clients for quite a number of years. Needless to say, these relationships were at the expense of the individual's financial health. Your success or failure is up to you and it's your responsibility to ensure your financial success.

When you choose an advisor, you must choose very carefully, and continuously analyze whether that advisor is carrying his or her weight and providing you with timely and accurate advice that specifically helps you to attain your financial goals. You are the quarterback of your financial plan, and it should be in harmony with your philosophy and your value system. You should try to find team members (advisors) that share your philosophy and that are committed to their profession and to excellence in their field. However, just as the quarterback knows what each of the team members duties and responsibilities are, you must also know the duties and responsibilities of each of your advisors, and you must always make the final decision as to the game plan to follow, even if you hire a financial planner as your coach.

Having worked for professional advisors over the years, I have come to the conclusion that most people choose professionals based on the wrong assumptions. The bottom line is you must hire a professional that can help you attain your financial goals and will commit himself or herself to give you accurate advice to help you to attain those goals.

To find professionals, I would suggest that you find friends and acquaintances perhaps in your field and ask them for referrals. Ask people that you respect and that appear to be financially successful, pragmatic, and intelligent, who they use for their professional advisors. Ask a number of friends so that you get a number of different professionals in order to interview them to hopefully help you achieve your goals. Once you get a list, call up the professional and ask that person to lunch or breakfast; and with a notepad in one hand and the following list of questions in the other hand (Professional Checklist of Questions), sit down with your advisor.

1. Describe your average client.
2. How long have you been in business? How long in this specialized or specific area?
3. How many other physician/clients do you have?
4. Do you have any one client who represented over 25 percent of your income in the last 12 months?
5. Do you plan on staying in this profession? How long?
6. Do you consider yourself an advisor or number cruncher?

7. What are your business/professional associations?
8. Can you give me 2 professional references to call regarding your character?
9. Can you give me 2 clients to call as references who have been clients for a few years?
10. How do you get most of your business? Referrals, purchase of practice, advertising, etc.?
11. What is your "ideal" client?
12. Why do you price that way?
13. If I decided your fee wasn't worth it and told you, how would you feel?
14. How much of my work will you do and how much will an associate do?
15. Have you ever been bankrupt?
16. Do you have business goals?
17. How do you run your business?
18. Do I have access to all documents in your file about my specific situation?
19. What assurances do I have of complete confidentiality?
20. How long has your staff been with you?
21. Do you like your job?
22. Are you one of those guys that reads professional journals at home while your spouse watches TV?

In addition to asking your investment advisor these questions, you should also ask him or her the following 3 questions:

1. What is your firm's investment philosophy?
2. Why do you charge fees only? Why do you charge fees and commissions?
3. What makes you better than the people down the street?

Your goal at this meeting should be to let him or her do all the talking and you just ask questions. Your prospective advisor should be so busy talking that he or she is halfway through with the salad by the time you have finished with your whole meal. That's all right, however, because when he or she becomes your advisor you should expect to have meetings when you haven't unfolded your napkin, and he is on dessert. When asking questions, do not be afraid to ask difficult ones, because difficult questions will get you the answers and the responses that will help you judge the character of the individual. For example, if you know that this advisor has gone through a divorce, say "Do you feel that you will stick around here now that you are divorced. . . or do you think you will move somewhere else for a new start" or "I hear that all your junior partners quit yesterday—why?" When you ask these questions, listen to the answers and watch the body language. If he or she hedges or gets uncomfortable answering your questions, ask follow-up questions that are specific to what made your advisor feel uncomfortable. Be merciless in asking questions, because you deserve the best and a good professional will respect you for your candidness and desire to hire the best.

What advisors will you need? To me, you will need six advisors to assist you with your financial plan. Although this does not mean that you will need six specific people to advise you, it does mean that you will need six specific areas addressed. These six areas are as follows: (1) legal work done by the attorney, (2) an accounting professional, (3) a financial planner that helps coordinate and advise you, (4) an investment advisor, (5) a retirement planning specialist, and (6) an insurance advisor, all of whom are often the same person as your financial planner or have other specialists within their firm working in these areas. Today you will often find an attorney in accounting offices that also may have specialists in the area of retirement planning or general financial planning.

Choosing a financial planner is one of the most important professionals you choose and you should find a financial planner that will address the whole of your financial situation and complement your other advisors. You should not hire a financial planner because he or she works for a large firm. You should choose a financial planner based first on his or her own individual credentials and secondly the back up services of the company.

Most financial planners are independent and although he or she may work for a reputable firm, it is very important that you have a very competent, knowledgeable, committed professional working for you. You should try to find a financial planner whose philosophy and attitudes mesh with your own. For example, in our company brochure we have our philosophy stated in writing for our prospective clients to see whether their attitudes are in harmony with our own. In addition to that we have a strong philosophy on investments. Our philosophy is it makes more sense to over diversify than to be under diversified.

Once in a while we get clients who do not like that idea. They say it is too much hassle to be overdiversified and they don't like getting reports on more than one or two investments. That's fine with us since we know that our philosophy works and that's what we feel comfortable with. That individual can go out and find someone that is possibly more in harmony with his philosophy. We also find that once in a while, prospective clients will only want to work with local investment advisors, trust companies, and trust services, and we use services from New York to California because we choose our advisors based on merit not on geography. However, often people will state that as a criterion and they may work with us as financial planners and let us coordinate the outside advisors, depending on the financial planner and the specific work that he or she does.

The financial planner may earn a fee for services, commission only for services, or a combination of fees and commissions. No one system is better than another. While the fee only financial planner will often say that "I am going to be much more objective because I charge a fee," the commission planner will say "The client is going to have to pay commissions to put an investment recommendation in order, so why not pay me a commission and I can be more reasonable on my fees or then I don't have to be paid a fee." While the fee and commission planner will say "I can lower my fees because I am also earning a commission." To me regardless of the way a financial planner is compensated, the most important decision is whether he or she can produce results and help you to attain your financial goals. I am not in favor of the financial planner's compensation system where they charge a substantial front fee in order to draw up a financial plan for you. To me, financial planning is long-term oriented and because tax laws, retirement planning laws, and nuances change often and since investment cycles and insurance policies and risk management techniques change over time, the financial planner should be compensated based on a relationship that will go on for many years, and not a slam bam great big fee or commission here's your plan type of system.

The relationship that you have with a financial planner will develop and grow over time, and the trust should come only after what your financial planner tells you will pass comes to pass. You should not be forced into a relationship because you paid a large fee or commission upfront and you feel that you want to get your money's worth. My feeling is that you should always be even with your financial planner and that he or she should be able to make the commitment to you to be compensated over a long-term approach. If you currently have an attorney, an accountant, an insurance agent, or an investment advisor that has worked with you over the years, and has given you very sound advice and whom you trust implicitly, and are going to be interviewing other advisors to assist you in finding a general financial planner, allow that trusted advisor to come to your luncheon meeting with that prospective financial planner or other advisor and let them shoot questions at that individual so that you make sure that you understand what that person can do for you and if that person is the right person for you. Often an objective third party can be very helpful. Another person that can be very helpful during your meeting is your spouse; since often the spouse can be watching the person's body language and could perhaps soften some of the difficult questions that you may have to ask. Make it so that your spouse also feels comfortable with that person as an advisor.

Each advisor will give you advice specific to certain areas in the financial arena. Following are the general characteristics and duties of each different advisor.

GENERAL ATTORNEY

A general attorney should help you with your real estate transactions and perhaps keep your minutes book together. Your attorney should advise you on simple will and trust arrangements, advise you on any contracts that you may enter into, etc. If your attorney has training in the area of tax, he or she could help you in analyzing the more complicated estate planning areas, looking at the tax structure of real estate or the other tax sheltered deals to assure that they should stand up based on current tax laws, etc. If your general attorney does not offer specialized tax services, then you should ask for a recommendation to an attorney that has that specialized knowledge. It is best to not force your tax attorney to do general legal work nor is it a good idea to make your general practice attorney do all of your legal work. For example, if you need to hire an attorney to protect you in a lawsuit, you would want the best trial attorney that you could find. Even though you may trust and respect your regular attorney, you should ask that attorney to give you a referral to a good quality trial attorney, if the case ever comes up. You should never hire a professional based on loyalty, but rather based on their ability to help you attain your goals.

ACCOUNTANTS

There are basically two types of accountants. There is an accountant that is a bookkeeper who basically takes the information that you give him or her and puts it down on pieces of paper so that you can file, for example, a tax return. These accountants are not advisors, and you should never force them into a situation of being advisors, since their main job is to take the numbers you give them and stick it on a piece of paper. This is not to say that that duty or job is not important; it is very important. However, do not expect your bookkeeper/accountant, even if he or she is a CPA, to be an advisor if their specific duties entail not giving advice, but merely putting your numbers down, although it may be a little bit neater than the accountant that works out of the basement of his or her house. A good accountant can also help you as an advisor. He or she should help monitor your income to make sure you do not get into a negative tax situation. He should review any tax strategy that may be recommended by your financial planner, investment advisor, realtor, or retirement planning advisor to assure that the specifics of that plan will help you. You should not have your bookkeeper review this information, but rather you should have your advisor accountant handle that duty. Many CPAs and accountants are getting very involved in the financial planning industry and this makes a lot of sense since many of them get very intimate with their clients and thus they are in an ideal situation to monitor the situation. A monitored situation, however, does not assure specific strategies will be recommended to help you achieve your financial goals. Do not force your accountant or CPA to give you specific investment advice about what types of investments to make. If they are not properly qualified and do not have lots of training in the retirement planning area make sure that you work with competent professionals in those areas. The retirement planning area is, as is the investment area, a specialized field and requires someone that has specialized training and time to devote to that area.

You may find it necessary to have a CPA, who gives you advice and reviews your situation, and a bookkeeper. However, it is often best to have your accountant also do the bookkeeping since he or she will then be able to monitor your situation and give you advice and make sure that you don't find out April 15 that you owe an extra $10,000 in taxes.

A good tax advisor will save you thousands and thousands of dollars in taxes, and to me a good tax advisor who is pragmatic and will spend some time learning about your situation is worth his or her weight in gold.

If your CPA has a CFP designation, keep in mind that CFP has six parts and only two parts have to do specifically with investment planning. Thus, a person with a CFP, or CLU or CHFC for that matter, does not have extensive training in the investment area specifically, because of having that designation. He or she may have lots of knowledge about investments, however, because of experience, training, or other specialized education.

INVESTMENT ADVISORS

Investment advisors come in all shapes and sizes and names. Some people consider their stock broker an investment advisor, some say their trust officer is an investment advisor, and some say you're not an investment advisor unless you work for a big institution and manage hundreds of millions of dollars for a mutual fund or large trust company. An investment advisor is any one that gives you advice regarding the allocation of your assets into any specific area. The branch officer of a bank when he or she sits down to tell an individual about their different CDs is acting as an investment advisor. An insurance agent that tells you to buy a whole life or universal insurance policy because the cash values will grow at a competitive rate of return is giving you investment advice, just as much as a stock broker who tells you to buy zero coupon bonds or an XYZ mutual fund in your IRA. My philosophy is that you want to be diversified, both in the types of investments and in the types of investment advice that you are receiving.

For example, if you want to allocate as part of a diversified portfolio 30 or 40 percent of your assets into common stocks, you should perhaps have 2, 3, or maybe 4 different investment managers managing that money. This can be done with a relatively small amount of money through the utilization of mutual funds. Many mutual funds will take $250 at no additional cost per dollar than a million dollar account, while you both get the same top notch, top drawer investment advice. Thus, if you have an IRA and you want to put half your money in common stocks, perhaps choosing two or three different good growth common stock mutual funds would make sense. Our clients will often have five or six different mutual funds or investment advisors involved in managing their portfolios. Often we hear that it would be much simpler to just choose one advisor. My answer is always no investment advisor is going to shine at all times. It usually costs no more to have a number of different advisors, especially through utilizing mutual funds or common trust, than it does to have one. I have received criticism from other professionals in my profession for this; however, their main criticism is how can I handle the accounting and bookkeeping of having a number of different advisors for even small IRA portfolios. My answer is "Don't you think it's worth it?" And their reply is "Yeah, but it's a hassle." We've worked out a relationship at our firm with a large trust company that does the trust accounting for us. Their fees are very reasonable and they allow us to have as many investments as we want in a trust account at no additional charge to our clients. Thus, it is no more expensive to have a number of different investments in the trust account than just having one.

The chapters on investments in this book should give you the good ammunition necessary to talk competently and intelligently with an investment professional or with your financial planner, so he or she will be able to recommend investment advisors who will fit your philosophies.

It is very important that your relationship with an investment advisor maintain an aloofness, so that if it becomes necessary to fire that investment advisor you are able to fire him or her if there is a changing of the guard or if their investment style does not seem appropriate for the economic cycles that you feel are coming. If you have trouble with the idea of firing an investment advisor, perhaps leave part of your portfolio with them and move the balance to another advisor. I have seen a number of cases where clients greatly damage their financial situations by sticking with a money manager who may have been great during one economic cycle who now is making havoc with their portfolio and jeopardizing their clients' financial well-being.

One manager who did extremely well in 1982 for our clients was fired in 1983 because we felt his style of investment would not be as favorable in the ensuing years. This was a difficult decision. It turned out to be very prudent, however, as this specific manager lost money for our clients who refused to move their money out of this manager's hands. If you are unhappy with the manager or think that changes need to be made you should communicate with him or her and if the investment firm he or she is with has other managers you may want to move the money to one of the different managers within that company. Finding one whose management style are perhaps more similar to your philosophy and what you think the economic cycles will be is very important.

Never be bothered by paying larger fees for investment advice and never judge an investment advisor based on fees, since a money manager who can make you 20 percent a year even after a 3 percent fee, is much better than a money manager that charges you a ½ percent, but only makes you an average 10 percent a year. Naturally the manager that has a higher performance may have substantially greater risk. However, this is not always the case, you must analyze the specific risk that each investment manager is taking on. Risk can be *quantitive* and there are many services that quantitate risk. Perhaps hiring a service to quantitate risk of the different managers would be helpful; however, generally you can tell the risk that a manager has by comparing his or her performance to a benchmark such as the Standard and Poor 500; if you're comparing common stock managers and then judging of the volatility around the Standard and Poor 500. For example, if one manager invests specifically in common stocks and earns 20 percent when the Standard and Poor is up 12 percent and loses 5 percent when the Standard and Poor is down 2 percent, while another manager just equals the Standard and Poor, you may want to hire the manager that had the greater performance since you are probably going to get more than your money's worth by hiring the manager with the superior performance.

INSURANCE ADVISORS

To me the ideal person to be a life, health, and disability advisor is your financial planner, if your financial planner is term oriented as illustrated in the chapter on insurance. It is very important that you find an insurance advisor whose philosophy is that insurance should be lean and mean to cover you adequately. You should hire an insurance advisor based on his or her philosophy meshing with your own. You should also make sure that your insurance advisor feels comfortable in having your account. Look at the specifics of how he or she chose to recommend any one policy over another to you. Your insurance advisor, just like any other advisors should be open to criticism and not shun it.

CASUALTY INSURANCE ADVISOR

The chapter on Insurance/Risk Management describes the different types of insurance you will need. It is very important that you have a good local insurance agent that can assure that you have properly managed and structured home, auto, liability, catastrophe and umbrella policies, etc. It is often best to have a casualty insurance advisor who is local, since when you have claims such as when the baseball goes through the front window or the lightning strikes the barn you may want to have a local agent who can make sure that your claims are handled properly and efficiently. Also make sure that your agent is aware of your ever changing situation so that when you put up the new satellite dish, a rider is added to your homeowners policy to cover your new property.

There are also other types of advisors that you will use such as bank trust officers, tax sheltered experts, realtors, etc. These advisors should be hired in a similar way that you hire the other professionals. Since these advisors are specialists and are not used in all situations, you must go to them with that specific goal in mind and make sure that they can achieve your specific goals. For example, if you are going to a trust office for trust services such as self-directed IRAs or pension plans, make sure that if you want them to do investment advice, you hire them as an investment advisor, if you merely want them to do the accounting, then you just want to make sure that their accounting system is cost effective and their account statements are readable.

Figure 20-1 shows the way that advisors sometimes work. As you can see, it can get very complicated and a good financial planner can help you to make things much simpler as illustrated on the bottom of Figure 20-1, called "The Easy Way If You Have A Good Financial Planner."

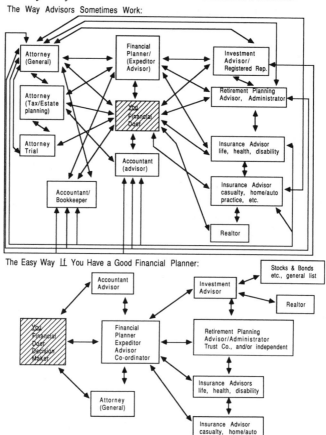

Fig. 20-1.

21
Developing a Financial Plan

The first chapters of this book dealt with giving you the knowledge and the philosophy to help you understand the different aspects in financial retirement, investment, insurance, and estate planning. The knowledge you have gained from reading this book is only worthwhile if you use it and develop a written plan of action to assure your overall financial success. The primary goal of this book is to help you to develop a plan of action so that you can ensure yourself and your family that you will be financially successful regardless of the financial environment and your circumstances.

From my experience, and I am sure that this is common among other financial planners, most people fail financially because they procrastinate. They let the weeks, the months, and the years go by and never develop a specific plan to ensure the attainment of their financial goals. These procrastinators find themselves with children to be educated and no resources; close to retirement with only a modest amount of assets; or because of the death of a spouse, entangled in a quagmire of legal and accounting muck because they failed to have a will and estate plan.

As you learned earlier, financial planning is arranging your assets and income to achieve specific goals, and involves:

1. Setting goals and prioritizing those goals.
2. Writing down your specific situation, i.e., your assets and income so you know what constraints you have upon which to build your financial plan.
3. Writing down a specific plan of action in order to ensure that you achieve your specific goals, i.e., setting up a retirement plan, properly situating your insurance program, having wills and trusts drawn up to ensure financial security, etc.
4. The most important step is taking action towards achieving your goals through actualizing the specific plan of action that you have written out for yourself through your own efforts, a financial planner, and/or other advisors.
5. Monitoring your situation to ensure that your situation is always up to date and consistent with current tax laws, investment cycles and your own goals, attitudes, and family situations.

With our own clients, we like to act as if we have a new client coming to us when we review their situation periodically. This assures us that our client situation is always up-to-date with the latest techniques, and changes in client attitudes.

In Chapter 2 you gave yourself a financial exam. You wrote down your specific financial goals and your specific situation. You should turn back to Chapter 2 and review your situation and your goals in light of what you have learned in this book, and then you should set goals for yourself on what you want to achieve. Table 21-1 lists questions that you ask yourself before you decide about a financial plan. From the answers in Table 21-1 along with the information you wrote down on your sheets in Chapter 2, you should be able to write your goals down and prioritize them. Do not pervert your priorities—make sure that you keep them consistent with your lifestyle, your philosophy, and your attitudes.

Your financial plan should be balanced—do not strap yourself financially by starting out gangbusters on that new retirement plan and then after 6 months decide that it is no "fun to fund" and stopping it completely because you burn yourself and your family out by not being balanced.

Table 21-1
Identifying Financial Goals

1. Insurance Program
   • What income would I want if I became permanently disabled?
   • What lifestyle would I want for my family should I die?
   • How much income would my family need to support that lifestyle?
   • Is my casualty coverage adequate?
   • Am I adequately protected against major catastrophes or litigation, no matter how remote the possibility?

2 Lifestyle
   • Do I wish to educate my children?
   • Do I want to retire?
   • What lifestyle would I want at retirement?
   • How can I reduce taxes and have more money to spend now and in the future?
   • Do I want a major lifestyle-oriented property (e.g., vacation home, boat, or airplane)?

3 Annual Review
   • Is my financial plan of action consistent with my current goals?
   • Have tax laws, family changes, or other factors made it necessary to modify my wealth accumulation program, wills, trusts, or insurance program?
   • Should I use a financial planner to assist me, or do I have the time, temperament, and abilities to coordinate my financial components to accomplish financial well-being?

From Financial & Investment Planning, Ltd., Suttons Bay, MI. With permission.

If you have a goal of security for your family and have a need for insurance then you should use the charts in the chapter on insurance to help you analyze that situation.

If you want to educate your children or retire, the chapters on education and retirement should help you analyze the best strategies towards attaining those goals.

Regarding your investment program you should be able to analyze it fairly reasonably after reading the chapters on investment and investment planning. You also should realize that you will not be able to do all of the work on your financial plan yourself and will most likely want to use outside advisors. A financial planner can help to actually do a lot of work that you are doing yourself, an attorney can help you with business forms, wills and trusts, and investment advisors can look over your existing investment portfolio to help you develop a portfolio strategy to assure financial well-being.

You will notice in this book that there is very little written about budgets and budgeting money. Budgets should be used to help you get a handle on your income and expenses, and they can help you figure out where your dollars go and from watching where your dollars go, you should be able to figure out some of your priorities. For example, if most of your money is going towards lifestyle and taxes, with very little towards wealth accumulation, you should realize that you probably will need to have a financial planner help you in setting up a good financial plan of action, since your attitudes are more lifestyle oriented, and probably not oriented towards addressing your financial needs. The financial planner should be able to help you (without affecting your lifestyle) accumulate wealth by reducing taxes, streamlining your insurance program, using different business forms (i.e., incorporating your practice), or other financial planning techniques.

If you live a balanced life, there should be plenty of money to provide you with an enjoyable lifestyle, educational funds for your children, retirement security, and an adequate insurance program. What I find often is that a client is overweighted in one area; perhaps his retirement plan is at the expense of his insurance program or his insurance program is improperly set up and harming wealth creation.

Once you have set your financial priorities you next address each priority with a pragmatic and realistic methodology. You must not allow anyone through bad advice to distort your priorities, since we are dealing with your attitudes, goals, and objectives and not those of your mother-in-law or golf buddy. You must stay consistent with your philosophy.

Figure 21-1 is a flow chart that illustrates how income is usually used. Notice in the flow chart that first your money goes towards living expenses, food and shelter, clothing, insurance, taxes, etc. Next your money goes towards protecting that income from death or emergencies such as making sure that you have enough life and health insurance if needed,

HOW TO ALLOCATE YOUR ASSETS TO MEET YOUR GOALS

Proper financial planning involves the allocation of your assets and income to accomplish your financial and personal objectives.

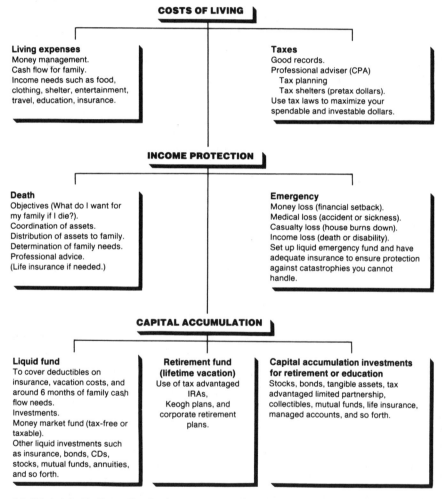

COSTS OF LIVING

Living expenses
Money management.
Cash flow for family.
Income needs such as food,
clothing, shelter, entertainment,
travel, education, insurance.

Taxes
Good records.
Professional adviser (CPA)
Tax planning
Tax shelters (pretax dollars).
Use tax laws to maximize your
spendable and investable dollars.

INCOME PROTECTION

Death
Objectives (What do I want for
my family if I die?).
Coordination of assets.
Distribution of assets to family.
Determination of family needs.
Professional advice.
(Life insurance if needed.)

Emergency
Money loss (financial setback).
Medical loss (accident or sickness).
Casualty loss (house burns down).
Income loss (death or disability).
Set up liquid emergency fund and have
adequate insurance to ensure protection
against catastrophies you cannot
handle.

CAPITAL ACCUMULATION

Liquid fund
To cover deductibles on
insurance, vacation costs, and
around 6 months of family cash
flow needs.
Investments.
Money market fund (tax-free or
taxable).
Other liquid investments such
as insurance, bonds, CDs,
stocks, mutual funds, annuities,
and so forth.

**Retirement fund
(lifetime vacation)**
Use of tax advantaged
IRAs,
Keogh plans, and
corporate retirement
plans.

**Capital accumulation investments
for retirement or education**
Stocks, bonds, tangible assets, tax
advantaged limited partnership,
collectibles, mutual funds, life insurance,
managed accounts, and so forth.

Note: This chart should not be considered legal or accounting advice. Seek competent professional help to assist you in accomplishing your financial goals.

Fig. 21-1. How to allocate your assets to meet your goals. (From Financial & Investment Planning, Ltd., Suttons Bay, MI. With permission.)

and third towards accumulating wealth for yourself or capital accumulation. Figure 21-1 is simplified; however, your first priority and commitment should be to your family to ensure their financial well-being should you die or become disabled. Then your capital accumulation goals would follow.

You will notice in our sample financial plan (see end of chapter) that the first thing addressed is Dr. Harold and Ann Waddell's estate and insurance needs. You should review the sample financial plan and see if any of the aspects and techniques used in this financial plan could be cloned and used in your own situation. You should use this as a guide to help you in setting up your own written financial plan.

If you plan on using a financial planner to help you in drawing up a financial plan, you should also review Dr. Waddell's financial plan to ensure that you are getting your needs addressed properly.

Many financial plans are 50 to 150 pages long. I find that digging through 50 to 150 pages tedious and counter productive. I think it was President Eisenhower who said "Give it to me on one piece of paper or don't give it to me at all." I think that the same can hold true with financial plans. A lot of financial planners are computer generated and basically 95 percent of the information in the financial plan is to make you feel like you are getting something for the money you paid. When you go to a dentist and he or she reviews your dental situation, he or she does not write up a long program. The dentist says, "You need that tooth drilled and that tooth filled and you might want to think about capping that tooth right there." He or she doesn't write you 3 pages on why it makes sense to fill that tooth and another 10 pages on why it makes sense to cap that tooth. He or she tells it to you specifically, concisely, and with enough information so that you can make a decision as to whether you feel that his or her ideas for your teeth make sense for you.

From my experience, I have found that writing the financial plan is the easy part for most people, especially if they are helped by a financial planner. The most difficult part of the financial planning process is doing it and consistent monitoring, to ensure lifetime financial success. On at least an annual basis you should formally sit down with your advisors to review your situation.

I have been working with people on arranging their financial, investment, retirement, and insurance programs properly for quite a number of years and have seen the results of proper planning. However, I have learned that reviewing the client's situation periodically to ensure that the situation is always in harmony with the client's goals, objectives, income, and attitudes, should be top priority.

Note in the sample financial plan that Harold and Ann Waddell appear to have no surplus money to go towards wealth accumulation. However, by properly arranging their debt they were able to free up $800 a month in nondeductible principal payments to go towards wealth accumulation. In their tax bracket this equates to being able to put away, toward accumulating wealth, about $12,000 with a cost, because of tax savings equal to the money currently going toward the nondeductible principal payments. Thus, Harold and Ann were able to put away $14,000 a year to more than adequately allow them to achieve their goals of educating their three children and income at retirement.

Rearranging debt service without saving that new-found cash flow can wreak havoc with your financial situation, since, if the money does not go towards building wealth, you are not building up liquidity and net worth to help achieve your wealth accumulation goals and will go backwards financially. If you do not have goals to accumulate wealth and plan on working for the rest of your life and never retiring, then rearranging your debt will help enhance your lifestyle now. However, I find that most people who do not have the goal of retiring may have the goal of having the "option of retiring."

It was noted in Chapter 1 that your most important investment is you and your practice. If you see opportunities where you could buy a new diagnostic machine that would increase your revenue and the profitability of your practice, you should put your money there first before you put it into retirement plans. If hiring a paraprofessional to assist you would make you more efficient and thus increase your income you should consider this before putting money in a retirement plan. Thus, your first goal should be to increase the wealth that is created from your practice during the hours that you work. After a while your practice will reach a point where you are happy with its ability to create substantial income for yourself and that is the time to start putting money away in retirement plans.

You may find that along the way to increasing your practice's income that it is already generating excess income and natually you should fund your retirement plans then.

I find that there is a tendency to put off financial planning among some fulfillment oriented people who say, "Sutherland, I'll work forever. I love what I do, I am a doctor, I don't want to hassle with all this financial stuff." Those individuals often have difficulty figuring out what their financial goals are. However you can, get started towards financial well-being even if your wishes are as nebulous as "I want to create wealth, I want to have more money to spend, or I want to insure economic security for my family and minimize taxes, etc." All those attitudes are good starting points towards getting on the road to a properly situated financial plan.

There are many helpful tables in the Appendix that you may find useful in diagnosing your situation.

In the introduction to this book there is a Middle Eastern proverb that goes "Blessed is the man who gives advice but a thousand times more blessed is the man that takes that advice and uses it." I hope you are able to use this book to help ensure financial success for yourself and your family. This book gave you the tools to build your financial well-being, but it is up to you to make your declaration of financial independence.

Sample Financial Plan

©**FINANCIAL & INVESTMENT MANAGEMENT GROUP**
PENSION SERVICE DESIGN, INC./FINANCIAL & INVESTMENT PLANNING LTD

Date _____9__/_____/___85___

Name Dr. Harold & Ann Waddell

Social Sec. #'s _____/_____

Date (s) of Birth Age 40 ____/_Age 35____

Children:

Name	DOB	Name(s)	DOB
John Age 10	___	Kimberly	Age 5
Nare Age 8	___	_____	___

Business Phone# _____

50% Practice
Personal Phone# Near Hospital in Medical Offic
Business Address Building with other G.P.'s
and Specialists

_____

Home Address_____

_____

Investment Assets

Cash/Checking & Money Fund(s) $ ___5,000.___
3 years @ $2,000./yr. in C.D.'s
Individual Retirement Account(s) ___7,000.___

Retirement Plans. I.R.A. only... _____

Limited Parnerships

(list separately)................ _____

Real Estate .... _____

Misc. Life Insurance .... _____

.... Net Cash Value .... ___6,000.___

Securities total 100/sh. mut. fund ___1,800.___

(list separately) 100/sh. Growth ___2,200.___
Medical
Lifestyle Assets

Personal Residence (cost in 1985) 125,000

Furniture/Appliances .... ___28,000.___

Automobile(s) 2 newer autos..... ___25,000.___

Personal/Jewelry, art, etc. .... ___5,000.___

Sail boat.................... ___8,000.___

Cabin & 10 acres on Swamp Lake ___38,000.___

Business Assets

Real Business Assets .... ___10,000.___

Goodwill Value.. Modest........ _____

Receivables................. ___42,000.___

....

Total Assets ....$ ___326,000.___

Income:
198__ Earned $_____
       Unearned $_____
       Total $_____

198__ Earned $_____
       Unearned $_____
       Total $_____

Present Year Estimate:
Earned $ 88,000. (Mrs. Waddell does books and helps
Unearned $_____ on Thursdays as receptionist &
Total $_____ is paid $7,000 annually.

Liabilities

Home Mortgage (Pymt. $ 950.) $ 75,000.
15 years left
Balloon Year_____ Interest 13%
*Swamp Lake Cabin @ 8%
Other Real Estate (Pymt. $ 250.) 10,000.
4 Years left
Auto(s) (Pymt. $ 212.) (14 %) 5,200.(3 Y
       (Pymt. $ 298.) (7.7 %) 9,500.(3 Y

.... _____

Notes Payable: (Pymt. $ 150.)
(Purpose Sail boat) 5,000.
Balloon Year 3½ Yrs. Interest 12%
Loan against receivables @.... 8,000.
prime + 1% ($200./monthly)

Total Liabilities_____ $ 113,700.
Total monthly payments
@ $2,060.
NET WORTH................. $ 212,300.

Expenses

Fed. & State Income Taxes...... ___20,000.___

Real Estate Taxes............. ___2,000.___

Investment Accounts.......... _____

Listed above: Debt service -
Mrs. Waddell's 1-year college ___3,000.___
to get teaching certificate.   ..

                              ___ ___ ___

....

Total........................ $ _____

PERSONAL ADVISORS:

Accountant _____Phone#_____

Address_____

Attorney _____Phone#_____

Address_____

Bank & Officer 3 banks & Credit Union

Casualty Agent _____Phone#_____

INCOME & TAX PLANNING

Is your income predictable? Yes _x_ No_____

Do you plan on changing your present work position in the future? Yes_____ No_X_

Do you have a line of credit? Yes_X_ No_____ Amount _$10,000._ Financial Institution Name .

Have you ever done any income tax planning? Yes_____ No_X_ If yes, please explain.

_____

TAX PLANNING VEHICLES (Please submit pertinent documents)

_X_IRA   _____Deferred Compensation Plan _____Tax Sheltered Custodial A/C

_____Retirement trust   _____Limited Parnerships   _____Others (Please list)

_____Interest Free Loans _____501(c)9 V.E.B.A. Trusts   _____

ADDITIONAL BENEFITS. (Please submit the pertinent documents.)

_____Salary Continuation Plan   _____Interest Free Loans

_X_Sick Pay/Disability $3,000. monthly after _____Company Car
                       30 days for 5 yrs.,
_____Health Insurance $1,000. monthly to age 65. _____Dues/Memberships

_____Medical Reimbursement Plan   _____Others (Please list)_____

_____Group Life Insurance   _____

If incorporated, date of incorporation: _____/_____/_____ Not incorporated.

Type of Corporation (P.C., Regular, or "Sub S")_____

FINANCIAL INDEPENDENCE INFORMATION

How much money do you estimate you need per month to provide for your basic living expenses (food, clothing, housing, entertainment, travel, etc.)? $_2,500._ + Taxes & debt service.

At what age do you wish to retire? _Be able to retire @ 60 if want to._

What do you feel that your investment assets should do for you? _Grow towards accomplishing goals of: 1) Educate children, 2) Build net worth, 3) Retirement security._

In terms of your assets directed to investment areas, please rate how you feel about the following statements:

	Strongly Agree	Agree	Disagree	No Opinion
A. Short term safety of capital is very important			X	
B. Longer term safety of capital is very important		X		
C. Inflation protection (maintenance of purchasing power) is very important		X		

Include some inflation hedges in Portfolio.

D. I am interested in pursuing **growth investments** and I'm willing to take the higher risks involved .... With some of my investments.

E. Income is very important to me.................. At retirement.

F. A balanced program of income and growth investments makes the most sense to someone in my circumstances.................. X

G. The idea of a professional manager assisting me in managing my investments to capitalize on opportunities and reduce risks through active management makes sense to me X

©FINANCIAL & INVESTMENT MANAGEMENT GROUP
PENSION SERVICE DESIGN, INC./FINANCIAL & INVESTMENT PLANNING LTD

I understand the cyclical nature of longer term investments. Yes__X__ No_____

CHILDREN'S EDUCATION

Have you considered setting aside money for your children's education? Yes__X__ No_____

If you, which levels of their education would you be paying for: Pre-college Yes_____ No__X__
Undergraduate Yes__X__ No_____, Post-graduate Yes_____ No__X__.

What percentage of your children's education do you feel should be paid for by the child through government loans, summer work, etc.? _____% Kids should pay for some with summer jobs.

Do you visualize any changes in your lifestyle upon your retirement? Yes__X__ No_____
If yes, please explain Travel more, want to live in Bahamas or Mexico in winter.

In "today's dollars", how much after-tax monthly income do you feel you will need upon retirement. $5,000. minimum.

FINANCIAL SECURITY NEEDS

What does financial security mean to you? Lower debt, more cash, security for my family if I die or get disabled.

If you were to become disabled before retirement, how much monthly after-tax income would you need to maintain a comfortable standard of living? $5,000./monthly.

Are there any unusual medical histories or financial circumstances that should be discussed regarding you or your dependents? All are healthy non-smokers.

How much money would you want in a highly liquid state such as a savings account for an emergency or opportunity reserve? $5,000. minimum.

Do you have Wills or related Trust Agreements? Yes__X__ No_____ If yes, when was the last time they were reviewed? 5 years ago – simple wills.

PRIORITIES

	TOP PRIORITY	PRIORITY	TO BE CONSIDERED
To reduce my personal income taxes	X		
To accumulate sufficient assets to provide an adequate after-tax retirement income		X	
To provide for my children's education		X	
To provide a monthly after-tax income of $4,000. + pay off debts. for my family in the event I become ill or disabled			
To build my net worth	For retirement and children's education.		
To arrange my affairs to minimize the impact of my death on my family		X	
To maximize the performance of my investment asset		X	

Other: Increase liquidity fund – may bring in partner in next 12 months, happy with office arrangement, would be able to get more space in building if brought in new partner or associate.

FINANCIAL & INVESTMENT MANAGEMENT GROUP
PENSION SERVICE DESIGN, INC./FINANCIAL & INVESTMENT PLANNING LTD

	Familiar With	Not Familiar With	Notes
Fixed Dollar Assets			
..ngs or C.D.'s	_____	_____	_____
.vings Bonds	_____	_____	_____
Money Market Instruments	_____	_____	_____
Government Securities	_____	_____	_____
Government Guaranteed Mortgages G.N.M.A.	_____	_____	_____
Deferred Annuities & Insurance Co. Products	_____	_____	_____
"Universal Life" (No or low-load products)	_____	_____	_____
Corporate Bonds	_____	_____	_____
Stock Market: (Individually managed or through mutual funds)			
Growth Stocks	_____	_____	_____
Blue Chip Companies	_____	_____	_____
Utilities & Income Stocks	_____	_____	_____
Option Writing	_____	_____	_____
Precious Metals & Collectibles	_____	_____	_____
Tax Favored Investments:			
Natural Resources	_____	_____	_____
Commercial Net Leased Real Estate	_____	_____	_____
Operating Real Estate	_____	_____	_____
Equipment Leasing	_____	_____	_____
Municipal Bonds	_____	_____	_____
Tax Deferred Annuities	_____	_____	_____
Tax Managed Trusts	_____	_____	_____

Notes:

Financial Planning Recommendations
for Dr. Harold and Ann Waddell

1. You should see an attorney to have your wills redone with a Trust arrangement to assure Mrs. Waddell and the children will have lifetime financial security. A Trust will:

   a. provide professional investment management of your insurance paid to the Trust;
   b. perhaps help reduce estate taxes at Mrs. Waddell's death.

   (Your attorney will advise you on the specifics of the use of Trusts as part of your overall financial plan.)

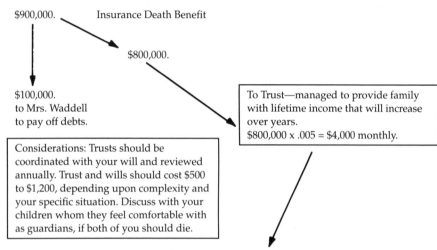

$900,000.   Insurance Death Benefit

$800,000.

$100,000.
to Mrs. Waddell
to pay off debts.

To Trust—managed to provide family with lifetime income that will increase over years.
$800,000 x .005 = $4,000 monthly.

Considerations: Trusts should be coordinated with your will and reviewed annually. Trust and wills should cost $500 to $1,200, depending upon complexity and your specific situation. Discuss with your children whom they feel comfortable with as guardians, if both of you should die.

$4,000. monthly to Family for income needs, education of children, etc. Hopefully, the trust investments will earn 6 percent and balance of earnings can be used to offset inflation.

Note: At Mrs. Waddell's death, money can go to children, charity, parents, etc., as desired.

2. a. See Insurance Schedule
      Dr. Waddell's Life Insurance Needs:
      $113,700. to pay off debts.
      + 800,000. to provide income.
      + 3,000. Mrs. Waddell' s college costs.
      - 17,000. Current liquid assets.
      $899,300. = Total insurance needed

      Ann's: $125,000. to pay off debts to free time and income for child rearing.

   b. Disability goal at $5,000. monthly. See Schedule.
   c. Re: Health Insurance—Upon review of your Health Insurance, it appears to be adequate.
   d. Your Casualty Policies should be reviewed to assure you are well covered; see your Casualty Agent and have him or her review raising your minimums and your deductibles.

3. Regarding Debt Structure

   Your debt structure should be rearranged for the following reasons:

   a. To free up cash flow to go toward wealth creation.
   b. To amortize debt over longer period to build up liquidity.
   c. Principal payments are not deductible and thus, in your tax bracket, you must earn approximately $1.60 to pay off $1. in principal.
   d. Inflation effects on your principal payments make it so that your principal payments in the future will be paid with $$'s with less purchasing power.
   e. You can accumulate wealth and net worth approximately two times as fast by redirecting your principal payment into tax favored retirement trusts.
   f. Only consumer debt for interest on your first and second home mortgage is 100 percent deductible. Debt for business purposes is also 100 percent deductible.

Current Debt Structure

Debt	Principal Amount	Monthly Payment	Amortization
Home	$75,000.	$ 950.	15 Yrs. left @ 13 %
Cabin	$10,000.	$ 250.	4 Yrs. left @ 13 %
Auto # 1	$6,200.	$ 212.	3 Yrs. left @ 13 %
Auto # 2	$9,500.	$ 298.	3 Yrs. left @ 13 %
Sail Boat	$5,000.	$ 150.	3 Yrs. left @ 13 %
Receivable Loan	$8,000.	$ 200.	Prime + 1 (4 ½ Yrs.)
	$113,700.	$ 2,060.	

Recommended Debt Structure

$113,700. Loan against home at 13% fixed - 30 years = $ 1,260. monthly.

Summary:

Current Debt Service @	$ 2,060.	
Recommended @	1,260.	
Net Savings @	$ 800.	to go toward Investment (through Retirement PlanTrusts.)

Note: Restructuring debt is dynamite—use with caution and save at least $800. monthly in a retirement plan.

4. Recommended strategies for wealth accumulation:

   a. Take wife off salary since she will no longer qualify for a tax deductible IRA and you will be able to put more into your pension plan.
   b. Set up a profit sharing plan retirement plan integrated with social security that allows voluntary nondeductible contributions (see plan specifics on next page).

5. Regarding Children's education

   You will have a substantial amount of wealth saved up in your Retirement Plan Trust and when your children are near college age, you could redirect part of your Retirement Plan contributions to:

   a. Hiring your children to do work around the office.
   b. Help get them started in a small business.

   Additionally you could:

   c. Tell them you will help them pay back their student loans.
   d. Get them a waitress or waiter job at your golf buddy's restaurant.
   e. Tell them to join the Air Force.

Note: Your goal currently should be to create substantial wealth and your #1 goal should be to put as much money into your tax qualified retirement plan as possible. If needed, this money can be used to help your children with college.

Recommended Portfolios, all in Self-directed Trusts

Dr. Sample's I.R.A.
@ Rollover of $7,000. in C.D.s
½ small companies' well-managed growth common stock mutual funds.
&
½ high yielding bond funds (through no front-end load mutual funds.)

Profit Sharing Plan
Initial Contribution of $6,000. - $2,000. — Government Guaranteed Participating Real Estate Mortgages.
$2,000. — Income Real Estate.
$2,000. — Income Leasing Partnerships.

Balance of Contributions
@ $1,000. monthly (dollar cost average)
$100. — International Common Stock Mutual Fund
$100. — International Bond Mutual Fund
$100. — Small Company Growth Mutual Fund
$100. — Gold Mining Shares Mutual Fund
$200. — High Yielding Bond Mutual Fund*
$200. — Government Bond Mutual Fund*
$200. — Growth/Income Common Stock Mutual Fund*

* To be managed by Portfolio Manager in a few years under "Market Timing" formula. After portfolio is to approximately $100,000. or so, start using individual securities in addition to mutual funds.

Note for this year: Since the year is ½ over, fund first 6 months from insurance cash values or sale of mutual fund or growth medical stock. If you like any of these investments, just re-buy them inside Retirement Plan Trusts.
(See below, Wealth Creation From Savings of $12,000 Annually at Various Rates of Return.)

Wealth Creation From Savings of $12,000 Annually ($1,000 Monthly) at Various Rates of Return

Annual Rate	0%	5%	8%	12%
12 Months	$12,000.00	$12,278.86	$12,449.93	$12,682.50
2 Years	24,000.00	25,185.92	25,933.19	26,973.46
3 Years	36,000.00	38,753.34	40,535.56	43,076.88
5 Years	60,000.00	68,006.08	73,476.86	81,669.67
6 Years A	72,000.00	83,764.26	92,025.33	104,709.93
8 Years B	96,000.00	117,740.51	133,868.58	159,927.29
10 Years	120,000.00	155,282.28	182,946.04	230,038.69
15 Years	180,000.00	267,288.94	346,038.22	499,580.20
20 Years	240,000.00	411,033.67	589,020.42	989,255.37

Present Life Insurance Program

Insured	Date	Policy Amount	Kind	Monthly Premium	Value	Net After Loans' Cash Dividends
Dr. Waddell	1969	$25.000.	Whole Life	$29.00	$2,000.	Yes
Dr. Waddell	1972	100,000.	Whole Life	85.00	2,500	Yes
Dr. Waddell	1980	150,000.	Annually Renewable & Convertible Term w/ Waiver of Premium during disability.	25.00	None	Yes
Dr. Waddell	1982	175,000	Term (as above)	28.00	None	No
Mrs. Waddell	1972	25,000.	Whole Life Family Plan	35.00	1,500	Yes
Children under Family Plan		2,000.	Term to age 21	Above		
				$202,000.	$ 6,000.	Included in Cash Values

Recommended Life Insurance Program

Insured	Date	Policy Amount	Kind	Monthly Premium	Comments
Dr. Waddell	New	$900,000.	Annually Renewable & Convertable Term w/ Waiver of Premium during disability.	$108.25	Policy could be converted to Adjustable Life in future if desired, which would build cash values. However, savings
Mrs. Waddell	New	$125,000.	Annually Renewable & Convertable Term w/ Waiver of Premium during disability.	$15.60	should be accumulated in tax qualified Retirement Plan.
John, Nate, & Kimberly	New	$10,000. + Guaranteed Insurability regardless of health to $250,000.	Adjustable Life w/Guaranteed Insurability & Waiver of Premium.	$6.00 (each)	Policies will build modest cash values; however, primary goal is guaranteed insurability benefit.

Present Disability Program

Insured	Policy Date	Amount	Monthly Premium	Cost of Living	Residual Benefit	Your Occupation Coverage
Dr. Waddell	1979	$ 1,000. Monthly for 5 years—	$ 25.	No	No	No
Dr. Waddell	1980	1,000. Monthly to age 65	55.	No	No	Yes
Dr. Waddell	1983	$ 1,000. Monthly for 5 years (after 60 days)	38.	No	Yes	Yes
		Total	$ 118.			

Recommended Disability Program

Insured	Policy Date Amount	Monthly Premium	Cost of Living	Residual Benefit	Your Occupation Coverage
Dr. Waddell	New $ 4,100. Monthly for life (after 30 days)		Yes @ 10% 6% Guaranteed	Yes	Yes—also, you are considered 100% disabled if
Dr. Waddell	New $ 900. Monthly to age Rider 65 (after 30 days) Offset by Social Security.	$310.01*	Yes @ 10% Guaranteed	Yes	your earnings drop to below 50% of your current income.

Notes: Receivables could be used to keep practice going for one month. Also, Dr. Friend said he would see Dr. Waddell's patients on his day off (Wednesday). (Office Overhead Expense Insurance does not appear necessary.)

* After liquidity is built up, change benefit period to 60 days, then 90 days to reduce premiums. Sixty day wait would cost $260.10 monthly. Ninety day wait would cost $ 240. monthly.

Dr. Waddell's Self-employed Profit Sharing Plan

Participant Allocation Schedule
(Integration Base $15,000.00; Contribution $14,517.04)

Name	Before Plan Compensation	With Plan Compensation	Allocation
Dr. Waddell	$ 95,000.00	$ 80,482.96	$ 12,000.25
Nurse Jane	$ 14,500.00	$ 14,500.00	$ 1,489.53
Part-time Physician's Assistant	not eligible	$ 0.00	$ 0.00
Receptionist Kim	$ 10,000.00	$ 10,000.00	$ 1,027.26
Employee total	$ 119,500.00	$ 104,982.96	$ 14,517.04

Notes: Plan covers only employees that worked over 1000 hours a year, are over 21, and have worked for the doctor for 1 year. Vesting schedule is year 1 = 0%, year 2 = 20%, year 3 = 40%, year 4 = 60%, year 5 = 80%, year 6 = 100%. Contribution is flexible and could be less than above if desired.

Cash Flow Effect of Setting Up New Plan

	Annually	Monthly
Contributions on behalf of doctor	@ 12,000	$ 1,000.00
Contributions on behalf of employees	@ 2,517	207.75
Total contributions to plan	@ $14,517	$ 1,209.93
Less tax savings @ 30%	- 4,355	- 362.93
Net cost/effect on budget	@ 10,162	$ 846.00

Note: If you have additional money, you can contribute to your profit sharing plan up to 15% of your after-contribution income or add a money purchase plan to your profit sharing plan. By properly structuring debt you can have $12,000 go toward wealth accumulation with an effect on your budget of only $46.00 ($846 - 800 = $46).

Steps to be Taken

1. See attorney and have wills and trusts revised.
2. Set up new insurance program (drop old insurance policies after new policies have been reviewed and are in force).
3. See bank about taking out mortgage of $113,700 to pay off present home mortgage, cabin, autos, sailboat, and receivable loan. (Save the difference in retirement plans.)
4. Take Ann off salary.
5. a. Set up new self-directed IRA and roll existing IRA to it or:
   b. Start Integrated Profit Sharing Plan (as illustrated) and fund it at $1,000/monthly.
   c. To fund Retirement Plans for this year sell mutual fund and 100 shares of Growth Medical and use insurance surrender values after new policies are issued.
6. See accountant and have quarterly taxes reduced because of retirement plan deductions.
7. Review your plan periodically. (The table below can work as a guide to assist you in reviewing your situation.)

Identifying Financial Goals

1. Insurance Program
   - What income would I want if I became permanently disabled?
   - What lifestyle would I want for my family should I die?
   - How much income would my family need to support that lifestyle?
   - Is my casualty coverage adequate?
   - Am I adequately protected against major catastrophes or litigation, no matter how remote the possibility?

2 Lifestyle
   - Do I wish to educate my children?
   - Do I want to retire?
   - What lifestyle would I want at retirement?
   - How can I reduce taxes and have more money to spend now and in the future?
   - Do I want a major lifestyle-oriented property (e.g., vacation home, boat, or airplane)?

3 Annual Review
   - Is my financial plan of action consistent with my current goals?
   - Have tax laws, family changes, or other factors made it necessary to modify my wealth accumulation program, wills, trusts, or insurance program?
   - Should I use a financial planner to assist me, or do I have the time, temperament, and abilities to coordinate my financial components to accomplish financial well-being?

From Financial & Investment Planning, Ltd., Suttons Bay, MI. With permission.

Appendix

Future Value Factors (F-1)

Years	1%	2%	3%	4%	5%	6%	7%
1	1.0100	1.0200	1.0300	1.0400	1.0500	1.0600	1.0700
2	1.0201	1.0404	1.0609	1.0816	1.0025	1.1236	1.1449
3	1.0303	1.0612	1.0927	1.1249	1.1576	1.1910	1.2250
4	1.0406	1.0824	1.1255	1.1699	1.2155	1.2625	1.3108
5	1.0510	1.1041	1.1593	1.2167	1.2763	1.3382	1.4026
6	1.0615	1.1262	1.1941	1.2653	1.3401	1.4158	1.5007
7	1.0721	1.1487	1.2299	1.3159	1.4071	1.5036	1.6058
8	1.0829	1.1717	1.2668	1.3686	1.4775	1.5938	1.7182
9	1.0937	1.1951	1.3048	1.4233	1.5513	1.6895	1.8385
10	1.1046	1.2190	1.3439	1.4802	1.6289	1.7908	1.9672
11	1.1157	1.2434	1.3842	1.5395	1.7103	1.8983	1.1049
12	1.1268	1.2682	1.4258	1.6010	1.7959	1.0122	1.2522
13	1.1381	1.2936	1.4685	1.6651	1.8856	1.1329	1.4098
14	1.1495	1.3195	1.5126	1.7317	1.9799	1.2609	1.5785
15	1.1610	1.3459	1.5580	1.8009	1.0789	1.3966	1.7590
16	1.1726	1.3728	1.6047	1.8730	2.1829	2.5404	2.9522
17	1.1843	1.4002	1.6528	1.9479	2.2920	2.6928	3.1538
18	1.1961	1.428	1.7024	2.0258	2.4066	2.8543	3.3799
19	1.2081	1.4568	1.7535	2.1068	2.5270	3.0256	3.6165
20	1.2202	1.4859	1.8061	2.1911	2.6533	3.2071	3.8697
21	1.2324	1.5157	1.8603	2.2788	2.7860	3.3996	4.1406
22	1.2447	1.5460	1.9161	2.3699	2.9253	3.6.35	4.4304
23	1.2572	1.5769	1.9736	2.4647	3.0715	3.8197	4.7405
24	1.2697	1.6084	2.0328	2.5633	3.2251	4.0489	5.0724
25	1.2824	1.6406	2.0938	2.6658	3.3864	4.2919	5.4274
26	1.2953	1.6734	2.1566	2.7725	3.5557	4.5494	5.8074
27	1.3082	1.7069	2.2213	2.8834	3.7335	4.8223	6.2139
28	1.3213	1.7410	2.2879	2.9987	3.9201	5.1117	6.6488
29	1.3345	1.7758	2.3566	3.1187	4.1161	5.4184	7.1143
30	1.3478	1.8114	2.4273	3.2434	4.3219	5.7435	7.6123
31	1.3613	1.8476	2.5011	3.3731	4.5380	6.0881	8.1451
32	1.3749	1.8845	2.5751	3.5081	4.7649	6.4534	8.7153
33	1.3887	1.9222	2.6523	3.6484	5.0032	6.8406	9.3253
34	1.4026	1.9607	2.7319	3.7943	5.2533	7.2510	9.9781
35	1.4166	1.9999	2.8139	3.9461	5.5160	7.6861	10.6766
36	1.4308	2.0399	2.8983	4.1039	5.7918	8.1473	11.4239
37	1.4451	2.0807	2.9852	4.2681	6.0814	8.6361	12.2236
38	1.4595	2.1223	3.0748	4.4388	6.3855	9.1543	13.0793
39	1.4741	2.1647	3.1670	4.6164	3.7048	9.7035	13.9948
40	1.4889	2.2080	3.2620	4.8010	7.0400	10.2857	14.9745
41	1.5038	2.2522	3.3599	4.9931	7.3920	10.9029	16.0227
42	1.5188	2.2972	3.4607	5.1928	7.7616	11.5570	17.1443
43	1.5340	2.3432	3.5645	5.4005	8.1497	12.2505	18.3444
44	1.5493	2.3901	3.6715	5.6165	8.5572	12.9855	19.6285
45	1.5648	2.4379	3.7816	5.8412	8.9850	13.7646	21.0025
46	1.5805	2.4866	3.8950	6.0748	9.4343	14.5905	22.4726
47	1.5963	2.5363	4.0119	6.3178	9.9060	15.4659	24.0457
48	1.6122	2.5871	4.1323	6.5705	10.4013	16.3939	25.7289
49	1.6283	2.6388	4.2562	6.8333	10.9213	17.3775	27.5299
50	1.6446	2.6916	4.3839	7.1067	11.4674	18.4302	29.4570

Note: 1% to 7% Future Value Factors (compounded annually). Used to figure how much value will increase at a stated % per year. Examples: $100. at 5% return per year will have a value in 5 years at $127.63. ($100. x 1.2763 = $127.63).

Future Value Factors (F-2)

Years	8%	9%	10%	11%	12%	13%	14%
1	1.0800	1.0900	1.1000	1.1100	1.1200	1.1300	1.1400
2	1.1664	1.1881	1.2100	1.3221	1.2544	1.2769	1.2996
3	1.2597	1.2950	1.3310	1.3676	1.4049	1.4429	1.4815
4	1.3605	1.4116	1.4641	1.5181	1.5735	1.6305	1.6890
5	1.4693	1.5386	1.6105	1.6851	1.7623	1.8424	1.9254
6	1.5869	1.6771	1.7716	1.8704	1.9738	2.0820	2.1950
7	1.7138	1.8280	1.9487	2.0762	2.2107	2.3526	2.5023
8	1.8509	1.9926	2.1436	2.3045	2.4760	2.6584	2.8526
9	1.9990	2.1719	2.3579	2.5580	2.7731	3.0040	3.2519
10	2.1589	2.3674	2.5937	2.8394	3.1058	3.3946	3.7072
11	2.3316	2.5804	2.8531	3.1518	3.4786	3.8359	4.2263
12	2.5182	2.8127	3.1384	3.4985	3.8960	4.3345	4.8179
13	2.7196	3.0658	3.4523	3.8833	4.3635	4.8981	5.4924
14	2.9372	3.3417	3.7975	4.3104	4.8871	5.5348	6.2613
15	3.1722	3.6425	4.1772	4.7846	5.4736	6.2543	7.1379
16	3.4259	3.9703	4.5950	5.3109	6.1304	7.0673	8.1372
17	3.7000	4.3276	5.0545	5.8951	6.8660	7.9861	9.2765
18	3.9960	4.7171	5.5599	6.5436	7.6900	9.0243	10.5752
19	4.3157	5.1417	6.1159	7.2633	8.6128	10.1974	12.0557
20	4.6610	5.6044	6.7275	8.0623	9.6463	11.5231	13.7435
21	5.0338	6.1088	7.4003	8.9492	10.8038	13.0211	15.6676
22	5.4365	6.6586	8.1403	9.9336	12.103	14.7138	17.8610
23	5.8715	7.2579	8.9543	11.0263	13.5523	16.6266	20.3613
24	6.3412	7.9111	9.8497	12.2392	15.1786	18.7881	23.2122
25	6.8485	8.6231	10.8347	13.5855	17.0001	21.2305	26.4619
26	7.3964	9.3992	11.9182	15.0799	19.0401	23.9905	30.1666
27	7.9881	10.2451	13.1100	16.7387	21.3249	27.1093	34.3899
28	8.6271	11.1671	14.4210	18.5799	23.8839	30.6335	39.2045
29	9.3173	12.1722	15.8631	20.6237	26.7499	34.6158	44.6931
30	10.0627	13.2677	17.4494	22.8923	29.9599	39.1159	50.9502
31	10.8677	14.4618	19.1943	25.4104	33.5551	44.2010	58.0832
32	11.7371	15.7633	21.1138	28.2056	37.5817	49.9471	66.2148
33	12.6761	17.1820	23.2252	31.3082	42.0915	56.4402	75.4849
34	13.6901	18.7284	25.5477	34.7521	47.1425	63.7774	86.0528
35	14.7853	20.4140	28.1024	38.5749	52.7996	72.0685	98.1002
36	15.9682	22.2512	30.9128	42.8181	59.1356	81.4374	111.8342
37	17.2456	24.2538	34.0039	47.5281	66.2318	92.0243	127.4910
38	18.6253	26.4367	37.4043	52.7562	74.1797	103.9874	145.3397
39	20.1153	28.8160	41.1448	58.5593	83.0812	117.5058	165.6873
40	21.7245	31.4094	45.2593	65.0009	93.0510	132.7816	188.8835
41	23.4625	34.2363	49.7852	72.1510	104.2171	150.0432	215.3272
42	25.3395	37.3175	54.7637	80.0876	116.7231	169.5488	245.4730
43	27.3666	40.6761	60.2401	88.8972	130.7299	191.5901	279.8392
44	29.5560	44.3370	66.2641	98.6759	146.4175	216.4968	319.0167
45	31.9204	48.3273	72.8905	109.5302	163.9876	244.6414	363.6791
46	34.4741	52.6767	80.1795	121.5786	183.6661	276.4448	414.5941
47	37.2320	57.4176	88.1975	134.9522	205.7061	312.3826	472.6373
48	40.2106	62.5852	97.0172	149.7970	230.3908	352.9923	538.8065
49	43.4274	68.2179	106.7190	166.2746	258.0377	398.8814	614.2395
50	46.9016	74.3575	117.3909	184.5648	289.0022	450.7359	700.2330

Note: 8% to 14% Future Value Factors (compounded annually). Used to figure how much value will increase at a stated % per year. Example: $1,000. at a 14% return per year—value in 50 years @ $700,233. ($1,000 x 700.233 = $700,233.).

Future Value Factors (F-3)

Years	15%	16%	17%	18%	19%	20%
1	1.1500	1.1600	1.1700	1.1800	1.1900	1.2000
2	1.3225	1.3456	1.3689	1.3924	1.4161	1.4400
3	1.5209	1.5609	1.6016	1.6430	1.6852	1.7280
4	1.7490	1.8106	1.8739	1.9388	2.0053	2.0736
5	2.0114	2.1003	2.1924	2.2878	2.3864	2.4883
6	2.3131	2.4364	2.5652	2.6996	2.8398	2.9860
7	2.6600	2.8262	3.0012	3.1855	3.3793	3.5832
8	3.0590	3.2784	3.5115	3.7589	4.0214	4.2998
9	3.5179	3.8030	4.1084	4.4355	4.7854	5.1598
10	4.0456	4.4114	4.8068	5.2338	5.6947	6.1917
11	4.6524	5.1173	5.6240	6.1759	6.7767	7.4301
12	5.3503	5.9360	6.5801	7.2876	8.0642	8.9161
13	6.1528	6.8858	7.6987	8.5994	9.5964	10.6993
14	7.0757	7.9875	9.0075	10.1472	11.4198	12.8392
15	8.1371	9.2655	10.5387	11.9737	13.5895	15.4070
16	9.3576	10.7480	12.3303	14.1290	16.1715	18.4884
17	10.7613	12.4677	14.4264	16.6722	19.2441	22.1861
18	12.3755	14.4625	16.8790	19.6733	22.9005	26.6233
19	14.2318	16.7765	19.7484	23.2144	27.2516	31.9480
20	16.3665	19.4608	23.1056	27.3930	32.4294	38.3376
21	18.8215	22.5745	27.0336	32.3238	38.5910	46.0051
22	21.6447	26.1864	31.6293	38.1421	45.9233	55.2061
23	24.8915	30.3762	37.0062	45.0076	54.6487	66.2474
24	28.6252	35.2364	43.2973	53.1090	65.0320	79.4968
25	32.9190	40.8742	50.6578	62.6686	77.3881	95.3962
26	37.8568	47.4141	59.2697	73.9490	92.0918	114.4755
27	43.5353	55.0004	69.3455	87.2598	109.5893	137.3706
28	50.0656	63.8004	81.1342	102.9666	130.4112	164.8447
29	57.5755	74.0085	94.9271	121.5005	155.1893	197.8136
30	66.2118	85.8499	111.0647	143.3706	184.6753	237.3763
31	76.1435	99.5859	129.9456	169.1774	219.7636	284.8516
32	87.5651	115.5195	152.0364	199.6293	261.5187	341.8219
33	100.6998	134.0027	177.8826	235.5625	311.2073	410.1863
34	115.8048	155.4432	208.1226	277.9638	370.3366	492.2235
35	133.1755	180.3141	243.5035	327.9973	440.7006	590.6682
36	153.1519	209.1643	284.8990	387.0368	524.4337	708.8019
37	176.1246	242.6306	333.3319	456.7034	624.0761	850.5623
38	202.5433	281.4515	389.9983	538.9100	742.6506	1020.6747
39	232.9248	326.4838	456.2980	635.9139	883.7542	1224.8097
40	267.8635	378.7212	533.8687	750.3783	1051.6675	1469.7716
41	308.0431	439.3165	624.6264	885.4464	1251.4843	1763.7259
42	354.2495	509.6072	730.8129	1044.8268	1489.2664	2116.4711
43	407.3870	591.1443	855.0511	1232.8956	1772.2270	2539.7653
44	468.4950	685.7274	1000.4098	1254.8168	2108.9501	3047.7184
45	538.7693	795.4438	1170.4794	1716.6839	2509.6506	3657.2620
46	619.5847	922.7148	1369.4609	2025.6870	2986.4842	4388.7144
47	712.5224	1070.3492	1602.2693	2390.3106	3553.9162	5266.4573
48	819.4007	1241.6051	1874.6550	2820.5665	4229.1603	6319.7488
49	942.3108	1440.2619	2193.3464	3328.2685	5032.7008	7583.6986
50	1083.6574	1670.7038	2566.2153	3927.3569	5988.9139	9100.4383

Note: 15% tp 20% Future Value Factors (compounded annually). Used to figure how much value will increase at a stated % per year. Example: $1,000. at 20% return per year—value in 36 years at $708,801.90 ($1,000. x 708.8019 = $708,801.90.).

Appendix

Time Value of Money—Future Value of $1 per Year (F-4)

Years	1%	2%	3%	4%	5%	6%	7%
1	1.0100	1.0200	1.0300	1.0400	1.0500	1.0600	1.0700
2	2.0301	2.0604	2.0909	2.1216	2.1525	2.1836	2.2149
3	3.0604	3.1216	3.1836	3.2465	3.3101	3.3746	3.4399
4	4.1010	4.2040	4.3091	4.4163	4.5256	4.6371	4.7507
5	5.1520	5.3081	5.4684	5.6330	5.8019	5.9753	6.1533
6	6.2135	6.4343	6.6625	6.8983	7.1420	7.3938	7.6540
7	7.2857	7.5830	7.8923	8.2142	8.5491	8.8975	9.2598
8	8.3685	8.7546	9.1591	9.5828	10.0266	10.4913	10.9780
9	9.4622	9.9497	10.4639	11.0061	11.5779	12.1808	12.8164
10	10.5668	11.1687	11.8078	12.4864	13.2068	13.9716	14.7836
11	11.6825	12.4121	13.1920	14.0258	14.9171	15.8699	16.8885
12	12.8093	13.6803	14.6178	15.6268	16.7130	19.1406	
13	13.9474	14.9739	16.0863	17.2919	18.5986	20.0151	21.5505
14	15.0969	16.2934	17.5989	19.0236	20.5786	22.2760	24.1290
15	16.2579	17.6393	19.1569	20.8245	22.6575	24.6725	26.8881
16	17.4304	19.0121	20.7616	22.6975	24.8404	27.2129	29.8402
17	18.6147	20.4123	22.4144	24.6454	27.1324	29.9057	32.9990
18	19.8109	21.8406	24.1169	26.6712	29.5390	32.7600	36.3790
19	21.0190	23.2974	25.8704	28.7781	32.0660	35.7856	39.9955
20	22.2392	24.7833	27.6765	30.9692	34.7193	38.9927	43.8652
21	23.4716	26.2990	29.5368	33.2480	37.5052	42.3923	48.0057
22	24.7163	27.8450	31.4529	35.6179	40.4305	45.9958	52.4361
23	25.9735	29.4219	33.4265	38.0826	43.5020	49.8156	57.1767
24	27.2432	31.0303	35.4593	40.6459	46.7271	53.8645	62.2490
25	28.5256	32.6709	37.5530	43.3117	50.1135	58.1564	67.6765
26	29.8209	34.3443	39.7096	46.0842	53.6691	62.7058	73.4838
27	31.1291	36.0512	41.9309	48.9676	57.4026	67.5281	79.6977
28	32.4502	37.7922	44.2189	51.9663	61.3227	72.6398	86.3465
29	33.7849	39.5681	46.5754	55.0849	65.4388	78.0582	93.4608
30	35.1327	41.3794	49.0027	58.3283	69.7608	83.8017	101.0730
31	36.4941	43.2270	51.5028	61.7015	74.2988	89.8898	109.2182
32	37.8690	45.1116	54.0778	65.2095	79.0638	96.3432	117.9334
33	39.2577	47.0338	56.7302	68.8579	84.0670	103.1838	127.2588
34	40.6603	48.9945	59.4621	72.6522	89.3203	110.4348	137.2369
35	42.0769	50.9944	62.2759	76.5983	94.8363	118.1209	147.9135
36	43.5076	53.0343	65.1742	80.7022	100.6281	126.2681	159.3374
37	44.9527	55.1149	68.1594	84.9703	106.7095	134.9042	171.5610
38	46.4123	57.2372	71.2342	89.4091	113.0950	144.0585	184.6403
39	47.8864	59.4020	74.4013	94.0255	119.7998	153.7620	198.6351
40	49.3752	61.6100	77.6633	98.8265	126.8398	164.0477	213.6096
41	50.8790	63.8622	81.0232	103.8196	134.2318	174.9505	229.6322
42	52.3978	66.1595	84.4839	109.0124	141.9933	186.5076	246.7765
43	53.9318	68.5027	88.0484	114.4129	150.1430	198.7580	265.1209
44	55.4811	70.8927	91.7199	120.0294	158.7002	211.7435	284.7493
45	57.0459	73.3306	95.5015	125.8706	167.6852	225.5081	305.7518
46	58.6263	75.8172	99.3965	131.9454	177.1194	240.0986	328.2244
47	60.2226	78.3535	103.4084	138.2632	187.0254	255.5645	352.2701
48	61.8348	80.9406	107.5406	144.8337	197.4267	271.9584	377.9990
49	63.4632	83.5794	111.7969	151.6671	208.3480	289.3359	405.5289
50	65.1078	86.1078	116.1808	158.7738	219.8154	307.7561	434.9860

Notes: Time Value Factors—used to figure what a stated amount of money will grow to per year. Future Value of $1. per uear (annual compounding). Example: $1,000. per year at 7% = $434,986. in 50 years ($1,000. x 434,986 = $434,986.).

Time Value of Money—Future Value of $1 per Year (F-5)

Years	8%	9%	10%	11%	12%	13%	14%
1	1.0800	1.0900	1.1000	1.1100	1.1200	1.1300	1.1400
2	2.2464	2.2781	2.3100	2.3421	2.3744	2.4069	2.4396
3	3.5061	3.5731	3.6410	3.7097	3.7793	3.8498	3.9211
4	4.8666	4.9847	5.1051	5.2278	5.3528	5.4803	5.6101
5	6.3359	6.5233	6.7156	6.9129	7.1152	7.3227	7.5355
6	7.9228	8.2004	8.4872	8.7833	9.0890	9.4047	9.7305
7	9.6366	10.0285	10.4359	10.8594	11.2297	11.7573	12.2328
8	11.4876	12.0210	12.5795	13.1640	13.7757	14.4157	15.0853
9	13.4866	14.1929	14.3974	15.7220	16.5487	17.4197	18.3373
10	15.6455	16.5603	17.5312	18.5614	19.6546	20.8143	22.0445
11	17.9771	19.1407	20.3843	21.7132	23.1331	24.6502	26.2707
12	20.4953	21.9534	23.5227	25.2116	27.0291	28.9847	31.0887
13	23.2149	25.0192	26.9750	29.0949	31.3926	33.8827	36.5811
14	26.1521	28.3609	30.7725	33.4054	36.2797	39.4175	42.8424
15	29.3243	32.0034	34.9497	38.1899	41.7533	45.6717	49.9804
16	32.7502	35.9737	39.5447	43.5008	47.8837	52.7391	58.1176
17	36.4502	40.3013	44.5992	49.3959	54.7497	60.7251	67.3941
18	40.4463	45.0185	50.1591	55.9395	62.4397	69.7494	77.9692
19	44.7620	50.1601	56.2750	63.2028	71.0524	79.9468	90.0249
20	49.4229	55.7645	63.0025	71.2651	80.6987	91.4699	103.7684
21	54.4568	61.8733	70.4027	80.2143	91.5026	104.4910	119.4360
22	59.8933	68.5319	78.5430	90.1479	103.6029	119.2048	137.2970
23	65.7648	75.7898	87.4973	101.1741	117.1552	135.8315	157.6586
24	72.1059	83.7009	97.3471	113.4133	132.3339	154.6196	180.8708
25	78.9544	92.3240	108.1818	126.9988	149.3339	175.8501	207.3327
26	86.3508	101.7231	120.0999	142.0786	168.3740	199.8406	237.4993
27	94.3388	111.9682	133.2099	158.8173	189.6989	226.9499	271.8892
28	102.9659	123.1354	147.6309	177.3972	213.5828	257.5834	311.0937
29	113.2832	135.3075	163.4940	198.0209	240.3327	292.1992	355.7868
30	122.3459	148.5752	180.9434	220.9132	270.2926	331.3151	406.7370
31	133.2135	163.0370	20.1378	246.3236	303.8477	375.5161	464.8202
32	144.9506	178.8003	221.2515	274.5292	341.4294	425.4632	531.0350
33	157.6267	195.9823	244.4767	305.8374	383.5210	481.9034	606.5199
34	171.3168	214.7108	270.0244	340.5896	430.6635	545.6808	692.5727
	186.1021	235.1247	298.1268	379.1644	483.4631	617.7493	790.6729
36	202.0703	257.3759	329.0395	421.9825	542.5987	699.1867	902.5071
37	219.3158	281.6298	363.0434	469.5106	608.8305	791.2110	1029.9981
38	237.9412	308.0665	400.4478	522.2667	683.0102	895.1984	1175.3378
39	258.0565	336.8824	441.5926	580.8261	766.0914	1012.7042	1341.0251
40	279.7810	368.2919	486.8518	645.8269	859.1424	1145.4858	1529.9086
41	303.2435	402.5281	536.6370	717.9779	963.3595	1295.5289	1745.2358
42	328.5830	439.8457	591.4007	798.0655	1080.0826	1465.0777	1990.7088
43	355.9496	480.5218	651.6408	886.9627	1210.8125	1656.6678	2270.5481
44	385.5056	524.8587	717.9048	985.6385	1357.2300	1873.1646	2589.5648
45	417.4261	573.1860	790.7953	1095.1688	1521.2176	2117.8060	2953.2439
46	451.9002	625.8628	870.9749	1216.7473	1704.8838	2394.2508	3367.8380
47	489.1322	683.2804	959.1723	1351.6996	1910.5898	2706.6334	3840.4753
48	529.3427	745.8657	1056.1896	1501.4965	2140.9806	3059.6258	4379.2819
49	572.7702	814.0836	1162.9085	1667.7711	2399.0182	3458.5071	4993.5213
50	619.6718	888.4411	1280.2994	1852.3359	2688.0204	3909.2430	5693.7543

Notes: Time Value Factors—Used to figure what a stated amount of money will grow to per year. Future Value of $1. per year (annual compounding). Example: $1,000. per year at 14% = $406,737. in 30 years ($1,000. x 40 x 406.737 = $406,737.).

Time Value of Money—Future Value of $1 per Year

Years	15%	16%	17%	18%	19%	20%
1	1.1500	1.1600	1.1700	1.1800	1.1900	1.2000
2	2.4725	2.5056	2.5389	2.5724	2.6061	2.6400
3	3.9934	4.0665	4.1405	4.2154	4.2913	4.3680
4	5.7424	5.8771	6.0144	6.1542	6.2966	6.4416
5	7.7537	7.9775	8.2068	8.4420	8.6830	8.9299
6	10.0668	10.4139	10.7720	11.1415	11.5227	11.9159
7	12.7268	13.2401	13.7733	14.3270	14.9020	15.4991
8	15.7858	16.5185	17.2847	18.0859	18.9234	19.7989
9	19.3037	20.3215	21.3931	22.5213	23.7089	24.9587
10	23.3493	24.7329	26.1999	27.7551	29.4035	31.1504
11	28.0017	29.8502	31.8239	33.9311	36.1802	38.5805
12	33.3519	35.7862	38.4040	41.2187	44.2445	47.4966
13	39.5047	42.6720	46.1027	49.8180	53.8409	58.1959
14	46.5804	50.6595	55.1101	59.9653	65.2607	71.0351
15	54.7175	59.9250	65.6488	71.9390	78.8502	86.4421
16	64.0751	70.6730	77.9792	86.0680	95.0218	104.9306
17	74.8364	83.1407	92.4056	102.7403	114.2659	127.1167
18	87.2118	97.6032	109.2846	122.4135	137.1664	153.7400
19	101.4436	114.3797	129.0329	145.6280	164.4180	185.6880
20	117.8101	133.8405	152.1385	173.0210	196.8474	224.0256
21	136.6316	156.4150	179.1721	205.3448	235.4385	270.0307
22	158.2764	182.6014	210.8013	243.4868	281.3618	325.2369
23	183.1678	212.9776	247.8076	288.4945	336.0105	391.4842
24	211.7930	248.2140	291.1049	341.6035	401.0425	470.9811
25	244.7120	289.0883	341.7627	404.2721	478.4306	566.3773
26	282.5688	336.5024	401.0323	478.2211	570.5224	680.8528
27	326.1041	391.5028	470.3778	565.4809	680.1116	818.2233
28	376.1697	455.3032	551.5121	668.4475	810.5228	983.0680
29	433.7451	529.3117	646.4391	789.9480	965.7122	1180.8816
30	499.9569	615.1616	757.5038	933.3186	1150.3875	1418.2579
31	576.1005	714.7475	887.4494	1102.4960	1370.1511	1703.1095
32	663.6655	830.2671	1039.4858	1302.1253	1631.6698	2044.9314
33	764.3654	964.2698	1217.3684	1537.6878	1942.8771	2455.1176
34	880.1702	1119.7130	1425.4910	1815.6516	2313.2137	2947.3412
35	1013.3757	1300.0270	1668.9945	2143.6489	2753.9143	3538.094
36	1166.4975	1509.1914	1953.8936	2530.6857	3278.3480	4246.8113
37	1342.6222	1751.8220	2287.2255	2987.3892	3902.4242	5097.3736
38	1545.1655	2033.2735	2677.2238	3526.2992	4645.0748	6118.0483
39	1778.0903	2359.7573	3133.5218	4162.2131	5528.8290	7342.8579
40	2045.9539	2738.4784	3667.3906	4912.5914	6580.4965	8812.6295
41	2353.9969	3177.7950	4292.0170	5798.0379	7831.9808	10576.355
42	2408.2465	3687.4022	5022.8298	6842.8647	9321.2472	12692.827
43	3115.6334	4278.5465	5877.8809	8075.7604	11093.474	15262.592
44	3584.1285	4964.2739	6878.2907	9530.5772	13302.424	18280.310
45	4122.8977	5759.7178	8048.7701	11247.261	15712.075	21937.572
46	4742.4824	6682.4326	9418.2310	13272.948	18698.559	26326.287
47	5455.0047	7752.7818	11020.500	15663.259	22252.475	31592.744
48	6274.4055	8994.3869	12895.155	18483.825	26481.636	37912.493
49	7216.7163	1043.4649	15088.502	21812.094	31514.336	45496.191
50	8300.3737	1210.5353	17654.717	25739.451	37503.250	54596.630

Notes: Time Value Factors—used to figure what a stated amount of money will grow to per year. Future value of $1. per year (annual compounding). Example: $1,000. per year at 20% = $470.981. in 24 years ($1,000. x 470.981 = $470,981.).

Examples of How to Use the Time Value Charts

Example 1: What is your real return to be on the Zero Coupon Bond that matures in 30 years at $ 100,000. and costs you $ 10,000. today? Go to Future Value Factor Table and look for 30 years—find number closest to "10." (10 x your money)—your approximate return would be "8%."

Example 2: You want to know what your $ 100,000. will grow to (in 10 years) if you add $ 10,000. a year and all your money earns 10%:

From Table F-2:

$ 100,000. x 2.5937 = $ 259.370.

From Table Y-2:

$10,000. (year) x 17.5312 = $ 175,312.

Add $ 259.370. to $ 175,312. = $ 434,682.

Example 3: You currently have $100,000. and you want to have $1,000,000. in 20 years—how much do you need to set aside annually if you earn 9%?

From Table F-2:

First—$ 100,000. x 5.6044 = $ 560,440.

$1,000,000. - $ 560,440. = $ 439,560.

(Goal—future value of current money you have.)

Need to fund for $ 439,560. more.

Go to Chart Y-2 (future value of $ 1. per year):

Find 20 years and 9% factor at $ 55.7645

$ 439,560. ÷ 55.7645 = $ 7,882.43

(Amount needed divided by factor = amount needed per year.)

Answer = $ 7,882.43 a year.

Check answer:

$ 7,882.43 x 55.7645 = $ 439,560.

$ 100,000. x 5.6044 - $ 60,440.

Total @ $ 1,000,000.

Amortization Table

Monthly payment required to pay off $ 10,000. debt at various rates of interest.

Years @	8%	9%	10%	11%	12%	13%	14%	15%
3	$ 313.37	318.00	322.68	327.39	332.15	336.94	341.78	346.66
5	202.77	207.59	212.48	217.43	222.45	227.54	22.69	237.90
10	121.33	126.68	132.16	137.76	143.48	149.32	155.27	161.34
15	95.57	101.43	107.47	113.66	120.02	126.53	133.18	139.96
20	83.65	89.98	96.51	103.22	110.11	117.16	124.36	131.68
25	77.19	83.92	90.88	98.02	105.33	112.79	120.38	128.09
30	73.38	80.47	87.76	95.24	102.87	110.62	118.49	126.45

Example: $10,000. loan at 12% over 20 years - payment + $110.11

$50,000 loan at 12% over 30 years = 5 x $102.87 = $ 514.35

1987 Individual Income Tax Rates

MARRIED FILING JOINTLY:

The tax before credits is-		The tax before credits is-		
Over	But not over	Flat Amount	+ %	Of excess over
-0-	$ 3,000	-0-	11%	-0-
$ 3,000	28,000	$ 330	15%	$ 3,000
28,000	45,000	4,080	28%	28,000
45,000	90,000	8,840	35%	45,000
90,000	—	24,590	38.5%	90,000

SINGLE TAXPAYERS:

The tax before credits is-		The tax before credits is-		
Over	But not over	Flat Amount	+ %	Of excess over
-0-	$ 1,800	-0-	11%	-0-
$ 1,800	16,800	$ 198	15%	$ 1,800
16,800	27,000	2,448	28%	16,800
27,000	54,000	5,304	35%	27,000
54,000	—	14,754	38.5%	54,000

UNMARRIED HEADS OF HOUSEHOLDS:

The tax before credits is-		The tax before credits is-		
Over	But not over	Flat Amount	+ %	Of excess over
-0-	$ 2,500	-0-	11%	-0-
$ 2,500	23,000	$ 275	15%	$ 2,500
23,000	38,000	3,350	28%	23,000
38,000	80,000	7,550	35%	38,000
80,000	—	22,250	38.5%	80,000

MARRIED FILING SEPARATELY:

The tax before credits is-		The tax before credits is-		
Over	But not over	Flat Amount	+ %	Of excess over
-0-	$ 1,500	-0-	11%	-0-
$ 1,500	14,000	$ 165	15%	$ 1,500
14,000	22,500	2,040	28%	14,000
22,500	45,000	4,420	35%	22,500
45,000	—	12,295	38.5%	45,000

1988 Individual Income Tax Rates

MARRIED FILING JOINTLY:

Over	But not over	Flat Amount	+ % Of excess over
-0-	$ 29,750	-0-	15% -0-
$ 29,750	71,900	$ 4,463	28% $ 29,750
71,900	149,250	16,265	33%* 71,900
149,250	—	41,790	28% 149,250

SINGLE TAXPAYERS:

Over	But not over	Flat Amount	+ % Of excess over
-0-	$ 17,850	-0-	15% -0-
$ 17,850	43,150	$ 2,678	28% $ 17,850
43,150	89,560	9,762	33%* 43,150
89,560	—	25,077	28% 89,560

UNMARRIED HEADS OF HOUSEHOLDS:

Over	But not over	Flat Amount	+ % Of excess over
-0-	$ 23,900	-0-	15% -0-
$ 23,900	61,650	$ 3,585	28% $ 23,900
61,650	123,790	14,995	33%* 61,650
123,790	—	35,501	28% 123,790

MARRIED FILING SEPARATELY:

Over	But not over	Flat Amount	+ % Of excess over
-0-	$ 14,875	-0-	15% -0-
$ 14,875	35,950	$ 2,231	28% $ 14,875
35,950	113,300	8,132	33%* 35,950
113,300	—	33,658	28% 113,300

*These rates include the 5% surtax to phase out the 15% rate for higher income taxpayers.

Federal Estate and Gift Tax Rates for After 1987

If the tax base* is-			The tax before credit is-	
0-	$ 10,000	0	18%	0
10,000-	20,000	1,800	20%	10,000
20,000-	40,000	3,800	22%	20,000
40,000-	60,000	8,200	24%	40,000
60,000-	80,000	13,000	26%	60,000
80,000-	100,000	18,200	28%	80,000
100,000-	150,000	23,800	30%	100,000
150,000-	250,000	38,800	32%	150,000
250,000-	500,000	70,800	34%	250,000
500,000-	750,000	155,800	37%	500,000
750,000-	1,000,000	248,300	39%	750,000
1,000,000-	1,250,000	345,800	41%	1,000,000
1,250,000-	1,500,000	448,300	43%	1,250,000
1,500,000-	2,000,000	555,800	45%	1,500,000
2,000,000-	2,500,000	780,800	49%	2,000,000
2,500,000+		1,025,000	50%	2,500,000

Note: Prior to 1988 the tax rate was higher on estates of over $2,500,000.

Unified Gift and Estate Tax Credit

Year of Gift or Death	Amount of Unified Credit†	Amount of Examption Equivalent
1981	$47,000	$ 175,625
1982	62,800	225,000
1983	79,300	275,000
1984	96,300	325,000
1985	121,800	400,000
1986	155,800	500,000
1987 +	192,800	600,000

Corporate Income Tax Rates 1988 and Beyond

Corporate Taxable Income	Rate on this Portion	Tax on this Portion
First $ 50,000	15%	$ 7,500
Next $ 25,000	25%	$ 6,250
Next $ 25,000	34%	$ 8,500
Next $ 235,000	39%	$ 91,650
Over $ 335,000	34%	—

* The tax base is the sum of the taxable estate and any adjusted taxable gifts made during life.
† If part of the former $ 30,000 gift tax exemption was used to shelter gifts made after 9-8-76, the credit figure in this column must be reduced by 20% of the exemption amount used.

Index